Nurse Manager

A Practical Guide to Better Employee Relations

2nd Edition

June Blankenship Pugh, MS, RN, CS
Consultant
Nashville, Tennessee

MaryAnn Woodward-Smith, MSN, RN, CS
Mental Health Clinical Specialist
Nashville, Tennessee

W.B. SAUNDERS COMPANY
A Division of Harcourt Brace & Company
Philadelphia   London   Toronto   Montreal   Sydney   Tokyo

W.B. SAUNDERS COMPANY
A Division of Harcourt Brace & Company

The Curtis Center
Independence Square West
Philadelphia, Pennsylvania 19106

Library of Congress Cataloging-in-Publication Data

Pugh, June Blankenship.
Nurse manager: A practical guide to better employee relations / June Blankenship
Pugh, MaryAnn Woodward-Smith.—2nd ed.

    p.   cm.

Includes bibliographical references and index.

ISBN 0–7216–6445–8

1. Nursing services—Administration.   2. Interpersonal relations.
  I. Woodward-Smith, MaryAnn.   II. Title.   [DNLM: 1. Nursing,
  Supervisory—organization & administration. WY 105 P976n 1997]

RT89.P84 1997   362.1′73′ 068—dc20

DNLM/DLC   96–28574

Nurse Manager: A Practical Guide to Better Employee Relations,
second edition   ISBN 0–7216–6445–8

Printed in the United States of America.

Last digit is the print number: 9   8   7   6   5   4   3   2   1

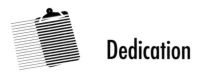

Dedication

To Jim and Gary,
who make our lives Wild and Wonderful!

Acknowledgments

*The pride of authorship can be surpassed only
by the pride of being the mothers of terrific
children—Jennifer, Janet, Ian, and Erin. We
are grateful for the blessing of their presence
in our lives and for all the encouragement they continue
to give us. Our special thanks goes to Ian,
President of U-R-My-Type, who worked tirelessly
and kept his positive attitude, even when he
couldn't read our handwriting.*

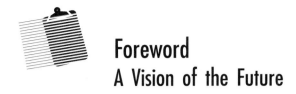

Foreword
A Vision of the Future

Managerial care is a whole new world for nurse managers. Old and new values are frequently in conflict as nurse managers strive for the correct balance between patient advocacy and cost-effectiveness. Adding to this complexity is health care's lack of awareness of itself as a service in the sense that a service is, in part, intangible and people-intensive. The value of the service is influenced by "value-added" interactions among patients and health care personnel.

With health care agencies focused on customer service, downsizing/rightsizing, and the increasing challenges of an appropriate staff mix, better employee relations and "managing the environment" are critical skills. Nurse managers at every level are in crucial frontline positions where patient and employee satisfaction intersect.

There is a need for practical, readable texts targeted for nurse managers, who come to their positions with a variety of educational backgrounds. Nurse managers must help nurses clearly state management goals and provide honest and timely feedback about why these goals are important and why nurses need to create win-win situations to meet these goals.

Frontline nurse managers serve as role models and greatly influence the environments of their units. Therefore, their use of cognitive restructuring and assertive communication techniques as discussed in this book can create an environment where stress can be reduced and employee and customer relations enhanced.

Nurse managers need to become more sensitive to the differences and inherent conflicts between their managerial roles and their clinical roles. This book stresses the need for nurse managers to avoid "taking care of" employees, to create support systems through networking, to establish power bases within the workplace, and to emphasize team-building with nonprofessional staff and interdisciplinary team members.

Nurse managers who utilize the skills presented in this book will create exciting, stimulating work environments where change will be seen as an exciting challenge, employees will feel good about themselves, and professional growth opportunities will abound.

COLLEEN CONWAY-WELCH, PHD, FAAN, FACNM
Professor and Dean
Vanderbilt University School of Nursing
Nashville, Tennessee

Preface
How To Use This Book

When we were writing the first edition of this book, we envisioned a manager feeling overwhelmed, frustrated, and discouraged. We saw her coming home and kicking back with a cup of hot chocolate and *Nurse Manager,* where she found practical solutions that she could use tomorrow. We have been gratified to hear reports of how many times our vision has become a reality. The publication of *Nurse Manager* began a wonderful adventure for us. We have had the privilege of traveling around the country, meeting health care providers, and validating our management philosophy. Because this simple, practical guide has been a success in the United States and Canada and has been translated into Japanese and Spanish, we have been encouraged to keep it current.

Current trends in health care delivery are making the management of other people a necessary skill for every nurse, not just those with the title of "nurse manager." Downsizing, outsourcing, restructuring, and especially the use of unlicensed assistive personnel are all placing heavier managerial burdens on registered nurses. In the current climate of restricted resources and cost-consciousness, failure to lead and manage effectively can seriously diminish the quality of patient care outcomes. Many nurses have not had a solid background in leadership and management as part of their basic education. Others may have a difficult time applying the broad spectrum of theoretical content learned in the classroom to the day-to-day realities they face in the workplace. This book will help nurses focus on the basic practical strategies needed to manage other people, to get them to do what needs to be done for safe, effective patient care.

In this edition we added new material and revised previous material based on our workshops and the current trends in health care. We have added chapters on time management, customer relations, and change. We are particularly excited about the changes in the chapter on stress management, which now includes the Seven Secrets of Stress Management. This is truly the last word on stress management.

Because we have learned that many staff educators and managers have used the first edition for inservice programs, we have included Creative

Teaching Tips at the end of each chapter. These tips will encourage group participation. If you are studying this material alone, use the Creative Teaching Tips as guides to increase your retention of the material. You will develop many of your own good ideas as you read this practical guide. Record them on the *That's A Good Idea* sheet (Appendix IX).

You may want to make this book the basis of an ongoing "Lunch and Learn." Study one chapter a month for a year. Have participants read the chapter and come prepared to discuss the content. Use the Creative Teaching Tips as a stimulus to start discussion. A group of managers could run this type of study group themselves, with the responsibility of facilitator rotating among the members.

When we think about changing behavior, we are reminded of a story:

> *A man is being chased by a tiger. As he comes to a steep cliff, the tiger is hot on his heels. His choices are to either jump or be eaten by the tiger. He jumps, but luckily there's a twig sticking out of the cliff and he manages to grab it. The tiger is leaning over the cliff, trying to get him. He can feel the tiger's hot breath on his neck, and he can see the jagged rocks below. Naturally the man resorts to prayer. He says, "Lord if you'll just get me out of this situation, I'll do anything you say." Out of the blue comes a booming voice, commanding, "Let go of the branch!" The man studies the jagged rocks again, looks up, and asks, "Is there anyone else up there?"*

You must be willing to let go of the branches of old behavior or ideas if you are to develop the skills required to be an effective manager. You've been asking for help with employee relations. Are you ready? Let go of the branch!

JUNE & MARYANN

Authors' note: We refer to managers as "she" throughout the book for ease of reading and because the majority of nurses are women.

Prologue
Once Upon a Time . . .

. . . Once upon a time in a large urban medical center, a group of health care providers got together for the purpose of developing a concise yet comprehensive list of skills that would serve as a guide to better employee relations. When they were finished, the group was proud of its work. "This is a very good list," said one of the nurse managers. "I wish more managers could see it." "Yes," agreed the director of nursing. "If all managers applied these skills, they would greatly benefit themselves, their employees, and their organizations." The hospital education director proclaimed enthusiastically, "Someone should write a book about these skills!"

And so someone did . . .

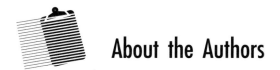

About the Authors

June Blankenship Pugh, MS, RN, CS, and MaryAnn Woodward-Smith, MSN, RN, CS, are clinical specialists in adult psychiatric and mental health nursing. They have years of experience in mental health, chemical addiction, women's issues, human relations, and staff development. They also offer continuing education programs nationally on topics such as leadership, stress management, assertiveness, and creative teaching.

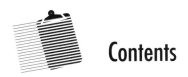

Contents

The Essential Skills

Chapter **1**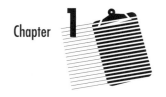

Assertive Management Style:
It's a Matter of Choice

Although there are other styles of management, assertive management offers the best way to feel good about yourself as a manager and the best way to help employees feel good about themselves and their jobs. In other words, an assertive management style promotes job satisfaction for both manager and employees. Assertiveness is a communication skill. Like perfecting a sport or mastering a musical instrument, it is a never-completed process. Practice makes us better, but change and circumstances present new challenges.

The following assessment will help you focus on some opportunities to improve your own assertive management skills. With your current management responsibilities in mind, read each statement and circle the response that applies to you most of the time.

Assertive Assessment for Managers

Yes	No	1. I would rather handle an unpleasant assignment myself than give it to an employee.
Yes	No	2. I have a hard time letting go of an argument.
Yes	No	3. When I try to be agreeable, the staff takes advantage of me.
Yes	No	4. I have difficulty letting someone do something his or her way instead of my way.
Yes	No	5. I agonize over reprimanding an employee or giving a bad evaluation.
Yes	No	6. I have a hard time saying thanks and showing appreciation to employees.
Yes	No	7. I bend over backwards trying to keep employees happy.

Yes   No   8. I tend to control meetings because I get impatient with people wasting time.

Yes   No   9. I find it hard to make decisions.

Yes   No   10. I tend to fly off the handle when the pressure builds.

Chances are you circled a few "yes" responses. These "yes" statements are opportunities to improve your assertive management style.

A Philosophy of Assertive Behavior

Our philosophy of assertive behavior is important for you to understand, because it lays a foundation for this book. It is as follows:

> **Assertive behavior occurs when an individual communicates personal choices that are in his or her own best interest while, at the same time, being respectful of others. Assertiveness is interpersonal communication that seeks "I win—you win" solutions. Assertiveness includes accepting responsibility for the consequences of personal choices.**

Examine carefully the following key components of this philosophy. Most likely you will find them thought-provoking.

Communicating

You communicate with every aspect of your behavior: what you say, how you say it, body language, dress, and the way you organize your surroundings.

Personal choices

You sort through countless options as you communicate. Every choice you make requires the rejection of choices you could have made. To the degree that you make these choices consciously, you have control over your communication. As you practice assertive skills, these assertive choices become automatic. You are like an accomplished musician who is conscious and in control of the music she is playing, but who has practiced until she plays the piece without thinking about each note.

In his or her own best interest

Assertive communication is usually associated with speaking up, taking action, and being open, honest, and direct. There are situations, however, in which it would be in your best interest to say nothing, to delay action, or to take no action. The key is to make this type of choice based on your best interest rather than on a fear of conflict.

Respectful of others

This implies a recognition of others and a regard for their feelings and vulnerability. Respect for others distinguishes assertive behavior from aggressive behavior.

I win—you win solutions

When you make choices that are in your best interest and that respect the feelings and choices of others, there is an opportunity for everyone to achieve some of what he or she wants. Assertive communication often involves negotiation and compromise, but it may simply involve recognition of and respect for everyone's feelings or opinions.

Accepting responsibility for choices

For every choice there is a consequence. Assertiveness means realizing that you have a great deal of control over consequences and events by the choices you make. Even when events happen outside your control, you can still choose your responses. Assertiveness also means not taking responsibility or credit for choices made by others.

The assertive manager firmly endorses the following assertive choices both for herself and for those under her supervision.

Declaration of Assertive Choices

1. I can choose to express my opinions and values, provided I do not set out to hurt others or to impose my opinions and values on them.
2. I can choose to state my own needs and priorities as a person regardless of what other people expect of me.
3. I can choose to ask for what I want or need.
4. I can choose to say "yes" or "no" for myself without having to offer justification.

5. I can choose to accept making a mistake and to assume responsibility for that mistake.
6. I can choose to change my mind.
7. I can choose to say "I don't understand" or "I don't know."
8. I can choose to decide for myself whether I am responsible for finding a solution to another person's problem.
9. I can choose to succeed and to accept responsibility for my success.

MANAGEMENT STYLES

The best way to understand an assertive management style is to compare and to contrast it with passive and aggressive management styles. While no one is always aggressive, passive, or even assertive, every manager has a pattern of communicating with employees that best defines her management style.

Assertive Style

Assertive health care managers place a high priority on producing results, but they also devote time and attention to the people needed to produce those results. Their goal is communicating with respect for their own rights and the rights of others. Consequently, they earn the respect of both their supervisors and their employees.

Aggressive Style

Aggressive managers are guided by a different goal. Their aim is to get what they and the organization want. Their priorities are clearly focused on results. For this reason they may be looked upon with favor by their organization until unhappy, disgruntled employees begin to request transfers. Because employees' needs are not a high priority, the aggressive manager does little to help them reach their full potential. Management by intimidation will never earn popularity or respect.

Passive Style

Passive health care managers aim for the goal of no conflict. Because they desire peace at any price, they place priority on what the employees want, often at the expense of producing good results. Although the organization may be displeased with the passive manager's inefficiency, employees will enjoy the manager's laid-back attitude. Eventually the passive managers will discover that they cannot always ensure everyone's satisfaction and happiness. Because these managers do not clearly communicate expectations or give performance-related feedback, employees do not have the opportunity to reach their full potential. In the passive manager's efforts to be well liked, she will never be well respected.

Contrasting Management Styles			
	PASSIVE	AGGRESSIVE	ASSERTIVE
OBJECTIVES	To avoid conflict	To get what I want	To communicate with respect
DESCRIPTION	Indirect Avoidant Placating Hypersensitive Rescuing	Blunt Invasive Insensitive Intimidating Domineering	Open Honest Direct Sensitive Enhancing
ACTION PRIORITIES	To meet the needs of the employees	To meet the needs of self and organization	To meet the needs of self, organization, and employees
SHORT-TERM CONSEQUENCES	Objective achieved	Objective achieved	Objective achieved
LONG-TERM CONSEQUENCES	Increased stress Decreased job satisfaction Decreased self-respect	Increased stress Decreased job satisfaction Decreased self-respect	Increased stress Increased job satisfaction Increased self-respect
INTERPERSONAL RELATIONSHIPS	May be liked but is not respected	Is not liked or respected	Is well-respected

Situation

At 11:45 A.M. Dr. Jones calls the charge nurse complaining that his diabetic patient, Mr. Smith, has not received foot care since admission 2 days ago. Dr. Jones is very angry. He demands that this oversight be taken care of before he makes rounds again at 3:00 P.M. The health care technician assigned to Mr. Smith is scheduled for lunch at noon. He is an active union representative.

Responses

Passive (no-conflict) Manager

The charge nurse is visibly upset by the phone call. Dr. Jones is certainly not someone she wants to cross. She dreads confronting the health care technician, who is always reminding her of his "legal rights."

Charge Nurse: Excuse me, Fred.

Health Care Technician (hurriedly): I know, it's time for me to go to lunch.

Charge Nurse: Well, yes, but, uh, Dr. Jones called. Well, uh, I know you've been busy, but have you had a chance to do Mr. Smith's foot care?

Health Care Technician: Nope! See you later. By the way, I'll be late getting back today. We've got a Union meeting at 12:30.

Charge Nurse: Well, uh, okay, I guess. *(Walks away talking to herself.)* I guess I'll do that foot care myself. It might be better for me to do it, anyway. I want to make sure it's done right.

In this example, the charge nurse achieved her goal. She avoided conflict and made the doctor happy. If you examine the long-range consequences, however, you will find that the charge nurse may have to deal with unpleasant side effects that were not a part of her goal. This charge nurse is paying a high price to avoid conflict. Chances are she feels resentful because no one appreciates her efforts to keep everyone happy. Because she tries to handle too much herself, she is overworked. She labors under a great deal of self-imposed stress, which will eventually take its toll on her physically if she does not leave the job first.

Aggressive (get-what-I-want) Manager

The charge nurse is angered by the phone call. She sets high standards, likes to keep the doctors happy, and views this report as an attack on her competency. She sees the health care technician headed for lunch. She approaches him with obvious anger.

Charge Nurse: **Where do you think you are going? I've been getting complaints about you all morning.**

Health Care Technician (defensively): **Who's complaining?**

Charge Nurse: **Never mind! Go do Mr. Smith's foot care! Now!**

Health Care Technician (angrily): **It's my lunch break and I've got a Union meeting at 12:30.**

Charge Nurse: **Patient care comes first around here. I want that foot care done before you go anywhere!**

Health Care Technician (stomps away talking to himself): **I'll bet that patient's been complaining about me!**

Charge Nurse (to herself): **You have to be tough with these people. Dr. Jones will be pleased.**

This charge nurse got what she and the doctor wanted—results. The charge nurse in this example is building resistance among her staff. Although she is interested in results, it will become harder and harder to produce the results she desires without the cooperation of her staff. When she pushes as hard as she can and uses all of her "big guns" to get the job done, what methods will be left for her to try? The stress of her job must also weigh heavily on her shoulders because, in a sense, she is carrying it all alone.

Assertive (communication-with-respect) Manager

The charge nurse checks the schedule and the patient to verify the information. She is annoyed that her colleague, Dr. Jones, has been put in this position. She is puzzled by the health care technician's poor performance.

Charge Nurse: **Fred, I see you're about to leave for lunch. I need to talk with you first.**

Health Care Technician: **I'm in a hurry. Remember, I told you about that Union meeting at 12:30?**

Charge Nurse: **Yes, I remember. Dr. Jones just called. He was very upset because Mr. Smith has not received foot care since admission. I checked the patient myself and I found Dr.**

Jones's report to be accurate. Looking at the assignment sheet, I see that Mr. Smith has been your patient since admission. Fred, I want to tell you how I feel. First, I feel angry because Mr. Smith's foot care was not done, and we both know how important foot care is for a diabetic. Second, I feel angry because I don't like having a colleague call me and report that a patient has not received proper nursing care. *(Pauses and touches employee's arm.)* You are much better than this. You usually pay close attention to these special treatments. Mr. Smith's foot care needs to be done before Dr. Jones makes rounds at 3:00 P.M. You haven't had lunch and you have a meeting at 12:30. What do you suggest?

Health Care Technician: I feel bad about this. I'll do the foot care now. I can take my lunch to the meeting.

Charge Nurse: Great. I won't give it another thought. I know I can depend on you.

The actions of this charge nurse were based on *A Philosophy of Assertive Behavior.* She was open, honest, and direct in her communication of negative feedback and expectations. She facilitated the employee's right to benefit the organization, and she allowed the employee to participate in resolving the problem. It is no accident that she has a spirit of teamwork and cooperation on her ward. The employees feel her concern for them, and they all work together to produce good results. This charge nurse experiences a lesser degree of stress and a greater degree of job satisfaction than the nurses in the two previous examples.

These examples illustrate that the assertive managerial response is the one most likely to have the desired results with the least undesirable long-range consequences. Being assertive will not guarantee success, but it will build your confidence and improve your odds for success.

Making Assertiveness Your Management Style

Assertiveness is not a talent. Assertiveness is a skill that is developed through practice. No one is born knowing how to be assertive. Having a knowledge of assertiveness is essential but is not enough. This book gives you the principles of being an assertive health care manager. Developing the skill will be up to you.

If assertiveness is a new skill for you or if management is a new role for you, you may want to create a peer support network where you can role-play assertive management techniques. You can also start practicing assertiveness in everyday occurrences with employees. Start with simple situations in which the outcome is not of crucial importance. Gradually work your way up to more complicated, critical situations. Just as with any skill, the more you practice, the more adept you will become at being an assertive nurse manager.

CREATIVE TEACHING TIPS

1. Have the participants affirm the *Declaration of Assertive Choices* by reading them aloud as a group.

2. Have the participants pair up with a colleague and rate each other using the *Assertiveness Assessment for Managers.* Critiquing management situations with a colleague will also sharpen their assertiveness skills.

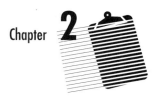

Assertive Verbal Skills:
Do You Say What You Mean?

There were two bachelor brothers, John and Joe, who lived in the country with their mother and an old cat. Now John and Joe never ventured out very much, but one day John decided he would go on vacation. John had never been away from home before, and the whole family's anxiety was high, but he promised he would call home every night and check on everyone. The first night he called home and talked with brother Joe. "Joe, how's Mama?" "Oh, she's fine, John." "Good. How's the cat?" "Well, John, I have terrible news. Mama and the cat went out on the road to get the mail, and a car came flying down the road, hit the cat, and killed him." John was naturally stunned. When he had recovered somewhat, he reprimanded his brother sternly: "Joe, that's no way to tell me bad news. You know how I loved that cat. You should have broken it to me gently. Tonight when I called home you could have said, 'Brother, the cat is on the roof, and we can't get him down.' The next night you could have said, 'Well, the cat fell off the roof, and we had to take him to the vet.' Then the third night you could have said, 'I'm sorry, John, the vet did all he could, but the cat died.' You see, that way you would be breaking the bad news to me gently." Joe apologized, "Well, okay, John. I'm sorry. I'll try to do better." The next night when John called home he asked cheerfully, "Hi, Joe, how's Mama?" There was a pause before Joe answered. "Well, John, Mama's on the roof."

We tell this story to illustrate the point that the words you choose are important. As a manager you are in a position of authority, and your position makes it even more critical to carefully consider your verbal communication. Some of the more difficult areas in employee communication are giving feedback, denying a request, dealing with criticism, and negotiating a compromise. You can learn some specific assertive verbal skills that will help you improve your communication in these areas.

"I" MESSAGES VERSUS "YOU" MESSAGES

Employees will be more receptive to your feedback when you phrase it as an "I" message. *"I" messages* take responsibility for one's own reactions, feelings, and needs (I think, I feel, I want). *"You" messages* imply blame and accusation (you said, you did, you should not have).

Practice turning "You" messages into "I" messages. Instead of saying to a staff nurse, "You never get to work on time," you could say, "I'm concerned that you are frequently late." Instead of telling a nursing assistant, "You know you cannot go to lunch until all the patients are fed," you could say, "I want you to make sure all the patients are fed before you go to lunch." Instead of saying to a doctor, "How do you expect anyone to read these orders? You're going to cause a nurse to make a big medication error one of these days!" you could say, "Please write your orders more legibly. I'm concerned that a nurse may make a medication error." Remember, "I" messages take responsibility for one's own feelings, whereas "You" messages cast blame on others.

FIRM PERSISTENCE

As a manager, there will be times when employees make requests that you will have to deny. Some managers find it difficult to say no; this is especially true for nurse managers, because nurses in their role as caretakers tend to be concerned about pleasing people. A technique that can be very useful in learning to say no is *firm persistence.* Calmly repeat over and over again what you want or what your position is until the other person agrees or gives up, or until you reach a compromise. Maintain a low-level relaxed voice when using firm persistence. You do not want to get into a shouting match.

Suppose you have an employee who wants the weekend off and you have to deny her request. The dialogue using firm persistence might go as follows:

> *Staff Nurse:* **I really need to be off this weekend. I just found out my family is coming from out of town, and I haven't seen them in 3 years.**
>
> *Manager:* **I can understand your feelings, but I can't give you this weekend off. What other options do you have?**
>
> *Staff Nurse:* **I just have to be off. They won't understand me working after they drove 1000 miles to see me.**
>
> *Manager:* **It sounds like a difficult situation, but I can't give you this weekend off. What other options do you have?**
>
> *Staff Nurse:* **Why can't you? I never ask to be off on weekends.**

I'm always willing to work and let other people have the weekends off.

Manager: **I appreciate your willingness to work in the past, but I can't give you this weekend off. Have you thought of any other options?**

Staff Nurse: **Please, I thought we were friends. I've done favors for you before.**

Manager: **I can certainly understand your disappointment, but I can't give you this weekend off. I'm willing to discuss other options.**

It is important to remember that it is not always necessary to respond to an employee's questions or comments. You simply maintain your position. What are the benefits of firm persistence? It puts you in control of the situation and keeps you from being manipulated. You do not have to spend time rehearsing arguments beforehand in order to be ready to deal with a conflictive situation. As with all assertive skills, you need to practice firm persistence until it becomes a technique you can use comfortably.

DEALING WITH CRITICISM

As a health care manager, you will have days when you feel that everyone is out to get you. Criticism is coming from all directions—doctors, your staff, administrators, patients, families, and visitors. The typical responses to criticism are increased anxiety and defensiveness. The following are assertive techniques that will help you avoid becoming anxious and defensive when being criticized:

Agreeing with the Possibility

Calmly acknowledge to your critic that there possibly is some truth in what he or she is saying. However, you remain the judge of your own behavior.

Staff Nurse: **I don't think the time schedule is fair.**

Manager: **Possibly it could be more fair.**

Asking for More Information

You acknowledge the criticism and clarify by asking for more information: what, when, where, and how?

> *Staff Nurse:* **I think you showed partiality in the time schedule.**
>
> *Manager:* **I'm sure I could have done a better job. What specifically did you notice?**

Owning up to the Mistake

You simply accept and acknowledge your own faults and mistakes.

> *Staff Nurse:* **Sue has had four weekends off in the past 2 months and I've had only one.**
>
> *Manager:* **You're right. I made a mistake. I'll look at the schedule and get back to you tomorrow.**

These techniques prevent situations from escalating, help you deal with manipulative criticism, and allow you to gain more from constructive criticism. Because the techniques decrease your anxiety and defensiveness, you become an approachable manager who is open and receptive to suggestions from employees.

COMPROMISE THROUGH ASSERTIVE NEGOTIATION

For a manager, the ability to reach a *compromise through assertive negotiation* is an essential skill. The best compromise is one in which all parties involved feel that they have, at the most, gotten all or some part of what they wanted. At the very least, they feel that their ideas, opinions, and feelings have been listened to and respected.

> *Staff Nurse:* **I would like 2 weeks off in June. I want to spend some time with my children while they're out of school.**
>
> *Manager:* **I can understand your desire to be off with your children this summer. I will be glad to give you some time off, but I can't give you 2 full weeks in June. I could give you a week in June and a week in July or August.**

Staff Nurse: **Okay. I'd like a week in June and a week in August.**

All compromises will not be as straightforward as this example. Each of us holds certain ethical and moral values that are important to us. Do not compromise if your self-worth or self-respect will be diminished.

CREATIVE TEACHING TIPS

1. Practice changing *"You" messages* to *"I" messages* and share examples (Appendix I).

2. Working in groups of three, role play *firm persistence,* techniques for *dealing with criticism,* and *compromise through assertive negotiation.* One person can serve as the observer or coach.

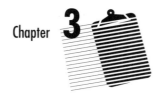

Nonverbal Communication:
Does Your Behavior Speak So Loudly They Can't Hear What You Say?

You often choose your words carefully in an attempt to elicit a favorable response, to be taken seriously, or to be understood correctly. You probably pay less attention to your nonverbal communication. Behavioral scientists tell us, however, that most of our communications are nonverbal; your employees respond mainly to your nonverbal language. Your carefully chosen words may be drowned out by the roar of your nonverbal behavior, of which you are often unaware. You can, however, develop nonverbal communication skills so that your body language becomes consistent with your words and actually reinforces the verbal message you are sending.

BEHAVIOR CUES

Your words may be assertive, but if your behavior gives a different message, then the listener will most likely respond to the behavior cues, and your verbal message will be ineffective.

For a dramatic illustration of the impact of nonverbal behaviors, make the following statement three times, changing only the nonverbal behavior to make the message passive, aggressive, or assertive. You can practice the statement in front of a mirror or with a friend, or you can use it as a role play to teach assertive nonverbal communication.

Statement

I am your new manager. I'm going to be meeting with each of you to set some mutual goals, so be working on some individual goals before our meeting. I will also be giving you frequent feedback on your performance.

Contrasting Nonverbal Communication Styles			
BEHAVIOR CUES	**PASSIVE**	**AGGRESSIVE**	**ASSERTIVE**
TONE OF VOICE	Timid, apologetic	Demanding	Confident
EYE CONTACT	Avoidant	Staring, intimidating	Comfortable, direct
GESTURES	Nervous	Threatening	Used for emphasis
FACIAL EXPRESSION	Tense, nervous smile	Tense, controlled	Relaxed, animated, friendly smile
POSTURE	Meek, humble	Rigid, tense	Comfortable, erect, confident
DISTANCE	Exaggerated, barricaded	Crowding, intimidating	Appropriate, considerate

Passive Nonverbal Behavior

The manager sits behind her desk or maintains an exaggerated distance from the employees. She is constantly examining and fumbling with a pen. She glances up occasionally but avoids making eye contact. Her facial expression is tense, with a nervous smile. Her voice is weak and the tone is apologetic. She hesitates frequently, and her statements often end with the inflection of a question, as if asking for approval. She giggles nervously.

Staff's reaction: What a pushover. No need to take her too seriously. Can't we get a real leader? She's going to give us feedback? Ha-ha!

Aggressive Nonverbal Behavior

The manager paces, walking up close to staff members with her hands on her hips or pointing at individuals. Her eye contact is steady and focused for a time on each individual. Her facial expression is tense and controlled. Her posture is rigid, and her voice is commanding. She speaks slowly with a tense jaw, pausing for effect and emphasizing each word.

Staff's reaction: Who does she think she is? Does she think this is the military? I don't think I'm going to like her or her feedback.

Assertive Nonverbal Behavior

The manager maintains a comfortable distance from the staff. Her desk is positioned so as not to present a barrier. Her hands are relaxed, either in her pockets or at her sides to be used for emphasis. Her eye contact is direct, moving from person to person. Her facial expression is relaxed and animated with a friendly smile. She maintains good posture and appears comfortable. Her voice is appropriately loud. She speaks clearly with a confident tone.

Staff's reaction: This sounds interesting. I'd better pay attention. She sounds like she means business. Maybe we can get something done around here now. I think she is someone I can respect.

It is important to point out that no single behavior makes a message aggressive, passive, or assertive. It is the total effect that is significant. You also need to identify the original intent or goal of the communication and determine if the behavior supports or nullifies that goal.

As an assertive health care manager, you want to have the respect of employees. You want them to take you seriously when you pass on information to them, and you do not want your nonverbal behavior to distract from or cancel out your verbal message. You want to project an image of self-assurance. Even when you are not feeling self-assured, you can, through developing these assertive verbal and nonverbal skills, appear more confident than you feel. The more confident you act, the more confident you feel; the more confident you feel, the more confident you act.

PROFESSIONAL IMAGE

Your appearance is an element of nonverbal behavior that makes a strong statement about you to others. It can be either an asset or a detriment in defining your role as a manager. You can reinforce your position as a manager through the way you dress. The lab coat is the status symbol of the health care professional. For men and women, a lab coat worn over a uniform or street clothes communicates authority. If you wear a uniform, choose the most business-like style possible. Be sure that your hair, shoes, and accessories also project a professional image consistent with your responsibility as a manager.

It is impossible to avoid creating an image through your dress and nonverbal behavior. You can choose to plan an image that will enhance your role, or you can choose to ignore the image issue. Choosing to ignore the issue may result in your having to work harder to overcome an image that is inconsistent with your managerial responsibilities.

CREATIVE TEACHING TIPS

1. Demonstrate the impact of nonverbal communication by saying the same brief statement three times to the group. Change only your nonverbal behavior. Ask for their reaction after each statement.

2. Suggest that participants watch a TV show without the sound and note the messages sent by the nonverbal communication, including the clothing.

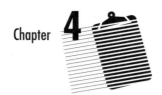

Chapter **4**

Managerial Listening Response:
Two Ears and One Mouth

"The Lord gave us two ears and one mouth. I guess that means He wants us to do twice as much listening as talking."

To listen more is good advice. As a busy manager, however, you must be concerned about using your listening time efficiently and effectively to benefit you, the employees, and your organization. You are already familiar with these assertive nonverbal listening behaviors:

- Use of frequent eye contact, while avoiding an anxiety-producing stare
- Adoption of a relaxed, receptive body posture
- Elimination of barriers, such as a desk, between you and the speaker

LISTENING STYLES

In order to be an effective listener, you must also respond to what you are hearing. Just as the style of your verbal and nonverbal communication can be identified as passive (no conflict), aggressive (get what I want), or assertive (communication with respect), your managerial listening responses can also be categorized according to these styles.

The following is an illustration of an employee with a personal problem and three different styles of listening responses by the nurse manager. Which response, in the long run, will be most beneficial to both the employee and the organization?

Situation

A staff nurse approaches the manager in the nurses' station.

Staff Nurse: **Helen, I've got lots of problems at home. You know my husband left me, and now that teenage son of mine wants to stay out all hours. I'm not sleeping well, and I feel so tired all the time I can barely drag myself to work. Yesterday I started crying when I was giving Mr. Richards his bath.**

Listening Response: Passive
(No Conflict)

Manager: **Oh, Claire, I'm so sorry. You know I'm always concerned about my staff. It was thoughtless of me to give you a heavy assignment. I understand how upsetting these family problems can be. I should be more supportive. Let's go in my office right now and talk about it. You probably need to get some things off your chest. Don't be concerned about your assignment. I'll ask someone else to cover for you. We'll talk as long as you need to. Now don't you worry because everything will work out just fine.**

The manager using this style of listening response is likely to spend more actual time listening than either of the other two. Quantity, however, does not necessarily equal quality. Because her goal is to avoid conflict, her listening is hampered by her heightened anxiety. Instead of focusing on the needs of the employee, she is focused on herself. She is more concerned about saying the right thing than about listening for the right thing. She places unrealistic demands on herself: "I should know the answer to all things." In an effort to be well liked, she has difficulty setting time or topic limitations with employees. She generally offers reassurance rather than an exploration of new ideas. Reassurance is safe and easy and makes the employee and the manager feel better for the moment.

Listening Response: Aggressive
(Get What I Want)

Manager (talking while still writing in chart): **Oh, I'm sorry to hear that. I'll tell you what I did when my husband left. I said, "Good riddance!" As for that teenager, I'd just remind him who is paying the bills. Tell you what, we've got a lot of work to do around here, but I can assign Mr. Richards to one of the other nurses since you're having so much trouble with men these days.**

This highly task-oriented and organization-conscious manager views talking as a waste of time, unless she is doing most of it. In order to meet her goal of getting what she wants, she is often too hurried and preoccupied to listen carefully. Like the passive nurse manager, she is focused on her own needs. Unlike the passive manager who is thinking, "I should," however, the aggressive manager is thinking, "I want—she should." After only half-listening, she decides what the employee's goals should be and even how she should feel. Frequently she cuts off an employee's expression of concern with a quickly formulated answer or rebuttal. She tends to minimize an employee's problems and feelings. Her responses are often characterized by detailed personal examples and unsolicited advice.

Listening Response: Assertive
(Communication with Respect)

> **Manager (puts down chart and gives employee full attention): It certainly sounds like you're going through some hard times right now. I'm glad you told me and I think we need to talk more. Let's meet in my office for about a half-hour right after you get back from lunch today. I'll get Elise to watch your patients for you during that time. I think I can suggest some resources that may be very useful to you.**

The time spent in listening by the assertive nurse manager is influenced by her attempts to maintain a balance between a concern for the employees and the needs of the organization. Whenever possible, she structures specific times for listening so that she can give the employee her full attention without interfering with the performance of duties.

Her self-confidence allows her to focus on the speaker and to actively process the information as she listens. She asks appropriate questions, both to obtain information and to help the employee solve problems. She realizes that employees must arrive at their own goals and solutions. She may choose to offer restrained, well-thought-out personal experiences that can be reassuring or can serve as models of behavior.

The assertive manager remains consistent in her role as a manager and avoids slipping into a counselor role. Any feedback given to employees is related to job performance. If the employee is experiencing personal problems, the assertive manager assesses the possibility of a crisis situation. She then proceeds to make appropriate referrals to assist the employee in the resolution of the problem.

CREATIVE TEACHING TIPS
1. Role play the three different listening styles and ask for critique from participants.
2. Ask participants to pair up and practice the assertive listening style.

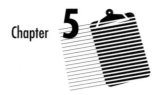

Chapter **5**

Stress Management:
The Final Word

STRESS IS IN YOUR HEAD

Stress is our body's reaction to our mind's assessment of a situation or event. Not only negative, unpleasant events create stress. Positive, happy events can create stress as well. The amount of stress we feel is in proportion to perceived threats to our status quo and perceived demands to adapt to change.

THE GOOD NEWS AND THE BAD NEWS

A key to managing stress is to realize that you have choices; therefore, you have control. You are both the captain and the navigator of your own boat. It is true that you cannot totally control life circumstances, and the water can be rough and full of hazards. After reading this chapter and applying the principles, you will have the equipment you need to survive. You will no longer float haphazardly, banging into rocks, getting stuck in brambles, flying over rapids, and dragging in the mud, never knowing exactly where you will end up and always dreading the next bend in the river. The good news is that you take control by the choices you make. You can avoid most hazards, you can lessen most collisions, and you can turn your boat back over when you capsize. You can chart your course and determine your destination. Even in a storm, you can survive. Before you get too excited, let us tell you that the bad news is that you are in control. When things don't go your way and people get in your way and you are in a terrible mood, you can no longer blame your mood on circumstances. You can still enjoy a pout, a fit, or a depression, but your mood does not come down on you like a thunderstorm. You are having this mood by choice. When you arrive at a port and it's not where you want to be, you can't blame luck. You can blame choice. You are responsible, not for all of life's circumstances, but for your responses to them. Consider this parable:

There once was a wise old man who lived in a country far away. Whenever the people of the kingdom had a problem, they would journey to the home of the wise man for an answer. His advice, if followed exactly, was always the right thing to do. His answers to the most complex questions were always correct. This resource was a great comfort to the adults of the kingdom. There were, however, two boys of that age and inclination to challenge all authority who decided they would ask the wise man a question that would be impossible for him to answer correctly. The first part of the plan involved catching a small bird. Then they quickly made a journey to the home of the elder and received an audience with him. While one of the boys held the bird behind his back, the other asked, "Wise old man, what does my friend have?" Not surprisingly, the old man answered, "A bird." "And, old man," taunted the bird's captor, "is the bird dead or alive?" If the old man answered "dead," the boy would open his hand and allow the bird to fly away. If the old man said "alive," he would crush the bird and drop it at the old man's feet. The two boys were trembling with excitement. For the first time ever, the wise man would be wrong! The old man's eyes were full of love and patience as he answered with a knowing smile, "The answer, my son, is in your hands."

TAKE CHARGE

You can manage your own stress by learning to manage your thinking. When you were born, you were blessed with the wonderful gift of a mind. When properly used, it is the only stress management tool you will ever need.

"Men are disturbed, not by things, but by the view they take of them."
Epictetus, first century A.D.

"Nothing is good or bad but thinking makes it so."
William Shakespeare

"Most men are as happy as they make up their minds to be."
Abraham Lincoln

"It is not the event, but rather it is our interpretation of it, that causes our emotional reaction."
Dr. Albert Ellis

All these words of wisdom are telling us that we can control our emotions and our stress if we learn to control our thinking. Dr. Albert Ellis, the pioneer of rational thinking, developed the following ABC model to explain how emotions occur:

A—*A*ctivating event

B—*B*eliefs (self-talk)

C—*C*onsequences (emotions and actions)

The sequence is literally **A→B→C.** Most people believe that events cause emotions and actions. If this were true, however, we would have no control over our emotions. Events and other people would determine our emotions and our stress level. The following example illustrates the **A→B→C** process:

Two 3-year-old children were playing with blocks in their den. A loud clap of thunder announced an approaching summer storm. One child ran crying to her mother. The other child laughed and continued to play. Both children heard the same sound. The difference in their reaction was due to their self-talk. One child said to herself, "I am scared. I could get hurt," so she ran to her mother. The other child said, "I like that noise. Do it again," so she laughed and began hitting two blocks together to mimic the sound.

If events determined our emotions and actions, then both children would have reacted in the same way.

Rational Thinking Reduces Stress

When you understand that you control your emotions and actions by what you think, you can learn to challenge your irrational thinking and to change it to rational thinking, thereby reducing your stress. Rational thinking is based on objective facts and helps us achieve our goals. The camera check is a technique recommended by Ellis for determining what is objective fact. Look at the situation as if you were looking through a camera lens. Facts are those things you can see through the lens void of any self-talk and emotion. Irrational thinking leads to negative choices that result in stress. The most common form of irrational thinking is *shoulditis*. We tend to *should* on other people and ourselves. *Shoulding* on others generates anger. If you tell yourself that someone else should have done something they didn't do, you generally feel angry. It is an irrational demand to say someone should do something. We do not have the power to make anyone do anything. We might prefer that someone do something and we might encourage her to do it, but we can't make her do it. When we *should* on ourselves, we create guilt. This is also irrational. If we didn't do something, we in fact didn't do it, and no amount of *shoulding* will change that. We can learn from the situation and choose to do it next time. *Should, must,* and *always* are words that make irrational absolute demands on self and others, thus generating anxiety and guilt. Eliminate these words from your vocabulary and use words such as *want, choose,* and *prefer.* For example, if you find yourself feeling like you must always be perfectly competent, remind yourself that it is impossible to always do everything perfectly. There are times you won't know the answer to a question or you'll make a mistake. No one is perfect. We all make mistakes. Believing you must be perfect creates anxiety within you, which increases the probability of mistakes and inhibits you from taking risks. It also leads to procrastination because you keep putting tasks off until you have time to do them perfectly.

Using the A→B→C→D Process to Improve Employee Relations

A. *A*ctivating event
   You are a new manager and one R.N. has come in 20 minutes late for the past three mornings. You talk with her and she says it won't happen again. The very next morning she is 20 minutes late.
B. *B*eliefs (self-talk)
   Your thoughts are, "I can't believe she's late again. Doesn't she think I mean business? I told her she had to be on time. She's doing this on purpose because I'm new. She thinks I won't do anything. She thinks she can get by with this. I'll show her. She can't treat me this way."
C. *C*onsequences (emotions and actions)
   You feel very angry and defensive. You yell at the R.N. in the presence of other staff members. You inform her that you will not tolerate this behavior and that you are going to write her up.

It is clear in this example that the manager's thoughts and beliefs about the situation resulted in irrational anger and inappropriate behavior. The manager could *D*ispute her irrational thoughts in the following way.

Irrational Thought: **Doesn't she think I mean business? I told her to be on time.**

Dispute: I need to find out what the problem is because we did discuss her tardiness yesterday.

Irrational Thought: She's doing this on purpose because I'm new.

Dispute: I don't know that for sure. She's been pleasant and helpful to me in other situations.

Irrational Thought: She thinks I won't do anything. She thinks she can get by with this. I'll show her.

Dispute: I need to talk with her and make sure she understands the consequences if she continues to be late.

Irrational Thought: She can't treat me this way.

Dispute: I have no evidence she is trying to "do anything to me." The only fact I have is that she was 20 minutes late.

Consequences of Disputing Irrational Thoughts: Although you are angry, you are not irrational. You calmly tell the R.N. that you want to talk with her in private after report. When you meet with her, you evaluate the facts, let her know how you feel about her behavior, and let her know the consequences if this behavior continues.

If you learn to **D***ispute* irrational thoughts, you can control your emotional reaction to conflict situations. When you are in control of your emotions, you can choose a more rational, assertive response. Remember, facts don't cause emotions. Your beliefs (self-talk) about situations cause emotions, and emotions lead to actions.

Seven Secrets of Stress Management

Based on the knowledge that the real secret to managing stress lies within controlling your thinking, we propose the following guiding principles. These principles are meant to guide your thinking in order to effectively reduce your stress.

1. I *choose to believe* that each person is doing his or her best.
Note the word *choose*. This is an attitude that allows you to reduce your stress in the immediate situation. It is not an evaluation of the behavior of other people. If you are in a supervisory capacity, it buys

you time to collect more information, to develop an intervention, and to formulate your feedback.

2. **Expectation affects outcome, so I *choose* to expect a positive outcome.**

   Positive expectations will open your eyes to possibilities and opportunities that are missed by people who expect negative results.

3. **If I always do what I've always done, I'll always get what I've always gotten.**

   If your behavior has been producing positive results, keep it up. If the results have been less than desired, you need to change your behavior.

4. **I can influence others, but only they can choose to change.**

   As both a health care worker and a manager, you are in the business of changing behavior, yet you do not have the power to make anyone change. Focus on what you can control. Work on your strategies to become a more positive influence.

5. **Life is not fair.**

   Do you believe life should be fair? When something negative happens, you may say "that's not fair" as if life were supposed to be fair. We have yet to find a person whose birth certificate guarantees that "life will be fair." For example, if life were fair we would either all be millionaires or all be in wheelchairs.

6. **Worry is more stressful than action.**

   You may often create stress for yourself by worrying about something instead of working on it. To decrease stress, take action. Get *around to it.*

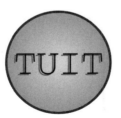

7. **I always have a *choice,* and all choices have consequences.**

   You are responsible for your own feelings and actions. For every choice you make there are consequences, so you need to look at your alternatives and choose the ones with the most positive consequences. You cannot control life circumstances, but you can control your reactions.

CHECK YOUR THINKING

To help you check your thinking when you are faced with a stressful situation, ask yourself the following questions:

1. What am I telling myself about the situation?
2. Is my self-talk in my best interest?
3. Is this situation my business?
4. Do I have the power to change the situation?
5. What are my alternatives in the situation?
6. What are the consequences of my choices?
7. What can I do *now* to reduce my stress?

The Seven Secrets of Stress Management are guaranteed to reduce your stress if you use them. Learn the Secrets by posting them prominently and reading them two or three times a day for 21 days (Appendix II). Psychologists tell us that if we practice something for 21 consecutive days it will become a habit. We recommend that you make two copies of Commitment to Reduce My Stress (Appendix III), sign it, and give a copy to a colleague. Make arrangements to touch base with your colleague at least twice a week to discuss your progress in applying the Secrets.

Using the Seven Secrets to Improve Employee Relations

The new health care manager in the previous example can use the Seven Secrets to reduce her stress so that she can more efficiently deal with the tardy R.N.

1. **I *choose to believe* that each person is doing his or her best.** Self-talk: *"I talked to her about tardiness yesterday, so there surely must be a good explanation for her being late again today. I'll listen to her explanation before I make a judgment."*
2. **Expectation affects outcome, so I *choose* to expect a positive outcome.** Self-talk: *"I will ask her what plans she has made to be here on time."*
3. **If I always do what I've always done, I'll always get what I've always *gotten*.** Self-talk: *"In the past this situation could ruin my day.*

Today I choose to keep things in perspective by practicing rational thinking and applying the Seven Secrets."

4. **I can influence others, but only they can choose to change.** Self-talk: *"I will continue to try to influence her behavior by making expectations and consequences clear. The ultimate responsibility is hers."*

5. **Life is not fair.** Self-talk: *"Although it seems unfair that I should have to take my time to deal with this employee's tardiness again, I realize it's just part of being a manager."*

6. **Worry is more stressful than action.** Self-talk: *"I'm going to deal with this situation as soon as possible and not let it distract me for the rest of the day."*

7. **I always have a** *choice,* **and all choices have consequences.** Self-talk: *"The employee has a responsibility to get here on time, and I have a responsibility as a manager to give her constructive feedback. We will both reap the rewards or face the consequences of our own behavior."*

CREATIVE TEACHING TIPS
1. Practice changing irrational statements to rational statements using Appendix IV.

2. In small groups, discuss the practical applications of the Seven Secrets (Appendix II).

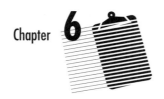

Chapter **6**

Are You Managing Time or Is Time Managing You?
Going for the Goal

Health care managers frequently have high expectations of themselves and of others. They often try to accomplish more than is reasonably possible in a given time. The nature and heavy responsibility of the job can lead to perfectionistic behavior and overidentification with their work. They often feel best about themselves when they are working hard. They may have a hard time relaxing and enjoying the pleasures of life. These traits can be summarized as the super-manager syndrome. How many of the following symptoms apply to you?

Super-Manager Symptoms Checklist

1. I do everything in a hurry.
2. I become impatient with others because they aren't working at my speed.
3. I do more than one thing at a time. For example, I read while eating, or I think about work while exercising.
4. I feel guilty when I am playing or relaxing.
5. I feel that everything I do must be perfect.
6. I believe that my worth is directly related to how much I accomplish.
7. I overschedule my time.
8. I become irritated when I have to wait in line or when I am caught in traffic.
9. I frequently feel too rushed to chat with a friend or to enjoy a beautiful sunset.

10. People often tell me that I need to slow down or to relax.

11. I find it difficult to ask for help, or I turn down help when it is offered.

12. I often put off starting a task because I won't have time to do it right or to finish.

If you endorsed any of these statements, it is possible that you are feeling worn out at the end of the day with few accomplishments and little satisfaction for the amount of energy you have expended. You may feel that your life is out of balance. Because you are working as hard as you can, what may be missing is an organized plan.

WISE INVESTMENT OF TIME

We all have the same number of hours to "spend" each day. Some people have a well-thought-out investment plan for their 24 hours that pays them big dividends in accomplishments and satisfaction. Others "nickel and dime" time away with very little to show for their investment.

If You Don't Know Where You Are Going, How Will You Know When You Get There?

Think of your life as a journey. First you have to decide on your destinations. Each of your many roles in life is a destination. Because this is your life journey, these are decisions that require an investment of time and collaboration with other travelers. This journey requires you to think beyond the limits of today and to project yourself into the future based on how you would like things to be. This can be called a mission statement, a philosophy of life, a vision, or a dream. It is a dynamic process. It is important to put your destinations in writing but not in concrete. Once you have decided on your destinations, you are ready to pull out the maps and travel brochures to decide on the places you want to visit along the way. You will want to do this planning for all the destinations or roles in your life. This chapter, however, focuses on your role as a health care manager. Goals describe the activities that will help you reach your destinations. Your goal-setting as a manager will fall into three categories:

1. **Organization Goals**

   The organization prescribes goals (policies) for which you will develop plans that you and your employees will follow. Sometimes even the plans (procedures) are defined by the organization and handed down to you to implement.

2. **Team Goals**

   Team goals are based on mutual team needs and interests of employees. When all staff members participate in determining the goals and in developing the plans, the process can be exciting. Traveling toward the destination becomes a team effort.

3. **Individual Goals**

   You and the staff have individual goals for professional growth. As a manager, you act as an adviser to staff and help them plan their own course of action involving work experiences, educational experiences, and career development opportunities.

Goal-Setting Steps

Many people fail to achieve goals because they never get beyond the "It would be nice if . . ." stage. A true goal is not just a wish, it has a plan of action and a deadline. As a manager, you are familiar with the quality improvement process. This same process can be used for setting organizational, team, and individual goals. In fact it is as easy **AS PIE:**

ASsessment: Determine a destination (desired outcome). Put the goal and action plan in writing.

Plan: Map out a route or action plan for getting there (steps leading toward achievement).

Intervention: Put the action plan into a time frame (overall and intermediate deadlines). Designate accountability (person or group responsible).

Evaluation: Keep current and on schedule (periodic review and revision).

If any one of these steps is missing, the goal-setting process is incomplete. Appendix V is a Goal-Setting Worksheet that outlines these steps. An example of a completed Goal-Setting Worksheet can be found on pages 67–68. Because the goals will be written and kept current, they become the basis of feedback and progress checks with employees. They will simplify the writing of employee evaluations and periodic unit reports.

Charting the Course

Successful travelers utilize only one calendar, a notebook-style time planner, which they keep with them at all times. The planner needs to contain a section for each of your roles in life. In each section you will write your evolving plans and the goals that move you toward your destination. Remember, each goal needs an action plan and deadline. Invest some time each week in planning your journey. When you ask yourself "What activities will move me forward toward my goals this week?" you will stay focused and make progress. You will arrive!

CREATIVE TEACHING TIPS
1. Develop a work-related goal using the Goal-Setting Worksheet (Appendix V).
2. Use a buddy system for sharing goals and for offering periodic encouragement toward the achievement of each other's goals.

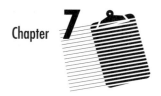

A Recipe for Creating a Team:
Together–Energized–Activated–Motivated

As a health care manager, you are designated leader of a group of people who represent a variety of educational backgrounds, skills, experience, personalities, levels of communication, and attributes. You have the responsibility of channeling all this diversity toward one outcome, that of excellent patient care. This outcome will happen only when you are able to create a **T-E-A-M**, a group of people who are:

> Together
>
> Energized
>
> Activated
>
> Motivated

The creation of this **TEAM** can be your most challenging, exciting, and rewarding experience as a manager. If you simply assign people to the same work area and expect them to be a team, however, it will be your greatest frustration and could even be your downfall. As the leader, you need to provide the climate and the ingredients for a **TEAM** process to develop over time.

CLIMATE CONTROL

As the manager on your unit, you are in charge of climate control. Rather than being a thermometer that merely reflects the prevailing climate, you can choose to be a thermostat and to exert some control over the climate. Your attitude is to a large extent reflected by the staff. Your behavior as a manager will influence the behavior of the staff. You serve as a role model, so model the behavior you expect. You need to have a positive visual image of the performance you expect from yourself as a manager as well as the performance you expect from employees. Engage in positive self-talk regarding this performance. For example, say to yourself, "Using my assertive communication skills, I expect that I will be able to assist each member of the staff to set goals and to become a more motivated, productive employee."

Within all employees there is a potential spark of excitement about their jobs. The manager with a highly developed **TEAM** has provided the proper environment for the spark to ignite into flames. Most employees want an opportunity to benefit the organization they work for and to reach their own full potential. The successful manager is creative in providing these opportunities for employees.

THE RECIPE FOR CREATING A TEAM

Most of us work for a salary. A familiar bumper sticker says it: "I owe, I owe, so off to work I go!" We know, however, that salary alone does not make work interesting or exciting and does not retain quality employees. There is a Recipe that a manager can use to create a great **TEAM** of **Together, Energized, Activated,** and **Motivated** staff.

Step 1. *Begin with the following ingredients: a clearly defined destination and specific measurable goals.* The staff can pull **Together** and focus their efforts when they understand the destination and the plan for getting there.

Step 2. *Blend with a larger cause or a group effort.* Each staff member can define how his or her personal contributions move the team toward the destination. They are **Energized** as they begin to see that a focused group effort accomplishes more than the separate individual efforts.

Step 3. *Serve with a feeling of accomplishment.* Because goals that are specific and measurable have been set, progress is easy to spot. You, the manager, are able to give feedback that will enhance individuals' self-esteem and self-confidence. The employee and the team will be **Activated** rather than stagnated.

Step 4. *Garnish with appreciation and recognition.* This step, more than salary, is the incentive that creates **Motivated** staff members. Be innovative and creative in ways to acknowledge individual and team effort. "Catch people doing good" (Appendix VII), thus rewarding and shaping desired behaviors. Be careful to be conservative in your praise, so that it will not lose its effectiveness. Expect employees to write self-evaluations and to give themselves credit for their own achievements.

The following are examples of what employees can accomplish when managers use the Recipe for Creating a **TEAM** and provide the proper climate for the goals to be accomplished.

1. The manager on Ward 8 North encouraged the staff to set a goal to win the hospital's poster contest for Hospital Week. All staff members submitted ideas for a theme, and she designated a committee to design the finished product. The committee agreed to work on the poster off duty, and the manager agreed to schedule 1 hour compensatory time for each member. The prize was a pizza party for all shifts. In addition, their poster was displayed in the hospital lobby.

2. When staff in a critical-care unit expressed concern about the resignation of two staff nurses who had been on the unit fewer than 6 months, the manager encouraged them to take some action. They set a goal to develop a plan that would help them better meet the needs of new employees. All staff were included in generating ideas, developing the plan, and implementing it when a new employee was hired for their area. At the end of 1 year, all vacancies had been filled, and there had been no resignations of new employees.

3. The manager at an adolescent chemical-dependence rehabilitation center formulated a goal that staff would be encouraged to become more involved in community education. She shared this goal with the staff, and they put together a program that included a skit and brief lecture aimed at helping parents teach their children to avoid drugs and alcohol. The staff contacted local schools, parents' groups, and other community organizations to offer prevention programs free of charge. They experienced a great deal of satisfaction from the appreciation expressed to them by those attending the programs. At the end of the year, the manager recommended to the center director that each staff member who participated receive a cash bonus.

Having no purpose or direction results in boredom and lethargy. Having clearly defined goals results in energy and action. As a manager interested in motivating employees, you need to set goals with employees, to give them feedback, and to use the power of your position to create challenging opportunities and supportive networks in which they can participate. Through your efforts, not only can employees meet the needs for which they were hired, they can also grow professionally and develop to their full potential. They will become **Energized, Activated,** and **Motivated.**

A TALE OF TWO MANAGERS

The main difference between leaders and followers is the leader's ability to have a vision of the future, to set goals, and to keep *herself* excited about these goals. In other words, as a manager you must continually **Energize, Activate,** and **Motivate** yourself. The following illustrates how utilizing the Recipe for Creating a **TEAM** keeps one manager a "Move-Ahead Molly," whereas failure to use the Recipe turns another manager into a "Burned-Out Betsy."

Move-Ahead Molly

Step 1. *Begin with the following ingredients: a clearly defined destination and specific measurable goals.* Molly has a clearly defined destination in each role of her life. She has formulated goals for herself, for her staff, and for her unit. Many of these goals have been generated from discussion with the staff. Molly's goals were developed from the following areas of interest:

A. Individual Professional Goals
   1. Increase research activity
   2. Keep work current (employee performance evaluations, for example)
   3. Keep work at work

B. Staff Goals
   1. Assist professional staff in becoming certified
   2. Increase staff expertise and responsibility
   3. Develop leadership skills in the professional staff

C. Unit Goals
   1. Provide adequate staffing on each shift
   2. Decrease absenteeism
   3. Develop a collaborative, collegial relationship between physicians and nurses

Step 2. *Blend with a larger cause or a group effort.* Molly is involved in working with other managers at her facility to provide a stimulating work environment for nurses as part of the hospital's recruitment and retention program. She is also part of a state nurses association work group to promote professionalism in nursing. This professional involvement outside her unit helps Molly keep perspective, prevents her from feeling isolated, and provides networking opportunities that enhance her career.

Step 3. *Serve with a feeling of accomplishment.* Because Molly has written goals, she is able to clearly identify her accomplishments. Her self-esteem and self-confidence are heightened.

Step 4. *Garnish with appreciation and recognition.* Molly receives recognition for her work because she is assertive in crediting herself for her accomplishments and because the positive results of her work are obvious. She is liberal in her praise and recognition of the staff.

Burned-Out Betsy

Step 1. *Begin with the following ingredients: a clearly defined destination and specific measurable goals.* Betsy probably has some goals in mind for herself, for the staff, and for her unit, but they are not clearly formulated or written down. Her goal each day is to get work done without a crisis. She is too disorganized to think in long-range terms and to involve the staff in goal setting.

Step 2. *Blend with a larger cause or a group effort.* Betsy is too busy getting the day's work done to attend nurse manager meetings or to become involved in hospital and professional committees that affect nursing.

Step 3. *Serve with a feeling of accomplishment.* Without written goals, Betsy is unable to identify her accomplishments.

Step 4. *Garnish with appreciation and recognition.* Betsy works hard putting out fires every day. She does little to distinguish herself; thus, she seldom receives recognition and frequently feels unappreciated. Rather than finding ways to praise and to recognize the staff, she sees them as her greatest source of frustration.

The following is a situation that any manager could face. As the example illustrates, however, using the Recipe allows you to successfully manage a stressful day and to create a **TEAM**.

Situation

> The manager reports for duty and finds a note from the night shift stating the coffee pot burned out. Two staff nurses call in sick, and two staff nurses are arguing. One threatens to go home if she has to work with "that nurse." Dr. Jane Smith interrupts the morning nursing report and asks to speak to the manager about a patient. The manager receives a call from the nursing office reminding her that five performance evaluations are due tomorrow. Checking her appointments for the day, the manager realizes that she has a lunch meeting with a staff nurse to discuss the nurse's goal to become certified. She also has plans to go out to dinner with her husband.

Burned-Out Betsy Reacts:

> "This is awful. I won't be able to handle all of this. This shouldn't be happening to me. It's not fair." She begins by checking out the coffee pot. She decides it cannot be repaired and makes plans to utilize her lunchtime to purchase a new one. She cancels her lunch meeting with the new staff nurse, telling the nurse that she will reschedule at a later date. She looks at her limited staffing schedule for the day and decides that she will have to be the medication nurse. During report she tells the two arguing staff nurses that she does not have time to listen to their dispute and she expects them to get on with their work. Anticipating a problem, she responds to the doctor's interruption by leaving report and spends 15 minutes talking to the doctor about the patient. She has two performance evaluations completed that she worked on at home last night. She was going to complete the other three at work today but decides she will have to take them home and do them tonight. She calls her husband and cancels their dinner plans.

Move-Ahead Molly Responds:

> This manager takes a few minutes alone in her office to review her priority list, which she made out the night before, and to check her calendar. She responds by thinking: "There's a lot going on here this morning. I can best handle it by being realistic about what I can accomplish, by setting priorities, and by delegating." Before going to report she notifies her supervisor that two of her staff nurses called in sick. The supervisor sends her one L.P.N. as a relief. She decides to let the L.P.N. give medications, and she assigns the two arguing staff nurses

to opposite sides of the ward. She asks each of them to come to her office at 10:00 A.M. in an attempt to identify and resolve their disagreement. When the doctor interrupts report, she explains that she will have the R.N. who is assigned to the patient meet with the doctor after report. She has been working on performance evaluations at work every day and has completed all but one. She has set completion of this one as a high priority today. She keeps the lunch appointment with the staff nurse to discuss her goal to be certified. She asks one of the staff to have the coffee pot checked out and to let her know what needs to be done. She leaves a message for the night shift that the problem is being resolved. She spends 1 hour working on her research project regarding empathy. Before leaving work, she checks completed tasks off her priority list and makes a new list for tomorrow. She calls her husband to confirm their dinner plans.

This example illustrates how two managers deal with the same circumstances. Even though Molly was faced with several obstacles as she began her day, she did not allow them to become roadblocks. As she stayed focused on her destination, she successfully maneuvered her way around, over, or through the obstacles and made considerable forward progress toward her goals. She was able to feel satisfaction at the end of a potentially stressful and frustrating day. Her confidence in her ability to meet the challenge of tomorrow was strengthened.

Betsy, on the other hand, self-destructed a little more. Because she had no defined destination or goals, she had no roadmap to give her a direction and nothing on which to focus. In fact, she took off in all directions, expending much more energy than Molly, with considerably less to show for her effort. At the day's end, she was tired and frustrated and was dreading tomorrow.

Both nurses began their careers with a desire to succeed. Molly has been able to move ahead, whereas Betsy tragically has burned out. If you are experiencing symptoms of burnout, you may wonder how you can rehabilitate yourself. The Recipe for Creating a **TEAM** is the answer. As you begin to formulate your destination and to set your goals, you will begin to feel excited about new possibilities. If you are having problems even thinking of goals, use the staff as resources. Brainstorming with them will not only generate new ideas but also stimulate everyone involved.

TEAM

As a successful manager, you are creating a climate conducive to growth. You are working to keep yourself moving ahead, and you are working *for* the staff to provide them with incentives to action. Your objective is to help yourself and the employees to benefit the organization and to reach full potential. Through your efforts you and the staff will become a **TEAM.**

Together

Energized

Activated

Motivated

CREATIVE TEACHING TIPS

1. Brainstorm motivational team-building ideas.

2. As a motivational exercise, work in groups on newspaper advertisements or television commercials ''selling'' the attributes of the organization or the team.

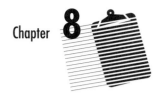

Feedback:
Staying on Course

Most managers would agree that feedback is essential in order to keep employees on course and to help them reach their goals. However, giving employees feedback is difficult for many managers. Effective managerial feedback can be defined as verbal and nonverbal communication with employees regarding their performance, based on mutually agreed upon goals.

THREE PURPOSES OF MANAGERIAL FEEDBACK

1. To help employees know how effective they have been in achieving their performance goals.
2. To direct subsequent behavior so that employees stay on course toward their desired goals.
3. To influence changes in employees' feelings, attitudes, perceptions, knowledge, and behavior.

SEVEN GUIDING PRINCIPLES

There are some basic principles to guide you as a nurse manager when you are navigating your employees toward your mutual goals. We call them the Seven T's of managerial feedback: Told, Timely, Timed, Targeted, Tactful, Truthful, and Tuned.

1. Told
   Inform employees that they will be given feedback regarding their performance. Feedback is best received when asked for, but at the very least it needs to be expected. Let employees know that they will

receive both scheduled performance evaluations and unscheduled, spontaneous feedback.

2. Timely

Positive behavior is more apt to be reinforced and negative behavior more likely to be corrected if feedback closely follows the behavior.

3. Timed

Be sensitive to an employee's particular circumstances and readiness to hear the feedback. If, for example, you know that an employee has just been informed of a personal loss, that is not the time to give her negative feedback about her performance.

4. Targeted

Feedback needs to be specific. When feedback is given in a general way, it is ineffective in reinforcing or in changing behavior because the employee does not know to which behavior you are referring. Try not to use judgmental words such as "good" or "bad." Give a description of the behavior in measurable and objective terms.

Avoid bringing up comments from past evaluations. Stay in the here-and-now. Relate feedback to performance goals. Avoid making critical remarks about an employee's personality. Make managerial feedback work-related and aimed at behaviors over which the employee has control.

5. Tactful

It is important that you make every effort to give feedback in such a way that it can be received without being a threat to the employee. If the employee feels threatened, she becomes defensive and cannot hear or make use of the information you are giving. Give feedback in a neutral manner. Use "I" messages and check your nonverbal as well as verbal behavior to make sure neither is aggressive.

6. Truthful

When giving feedback, you need to be open, honest, and direct regarding your feelings. Effective feedback is motivated by a desire to help the employee, not by a desire to satisfy your own need to express your feelings.

7. Tuned

Check feedback to ensure clear communication. Have the employee rephrase the feedback to see whether she heard your intended message. Because many people lack skills in receiving feedback they may distort your message.

TYPES OF FEEDBACK

There are two types of feedback: *positive,* which gives the message "You are right on course. Keep it up!" and *negative,* which gives the message "You're off course. Adjust." Contrary to what you might expect, most managers give negative feedback more freely than positive feedback. They tend to ignore employees when they are doing a good job and really let them have it when they make a mistake. They operate under the no-news-is-good-news philosophy. This approach does not help employees reach their full potential. It discourages risk taking and stifles creativity. Positive feedback, on the other hand, is encouraging. It stimulates people to strive to do even better.

Positive Feedback

*We observed a beautiful example of positive feedback between a 3-year-old boy and his 8-month-old sister. Big brother was very eager for his little sister to learn to crawl and to play with him in his room. The sister was at the doorway of her brother's room one morning, rocking back and forth on all fours, getting ready to crawl. Her big brother saw her and went running to her. He immediately started coaching her to crawl. From the next room we could hear him saying, "You can do it, Sis. I know you can. Come on."
We could hear his sister giggle with delight at the attention and encouraging words.* (How do you think your employees would react if you let them know that you notice their efforts, even in the beginning stages, and believe in them and their ability to do a good job?) *We looked around the corner at them and saw the big brother get on his hands and knees and proceed to show his sister how to crawl* (modeled behavior). *"See, this is the way to do it. Come on. There's lots of toys in my room. I'll let you play with them."* (Wouldn't it be great if you gave employees this kind of personal assistance and incentive when they're struggling with a difficult task?) *The sister continued rocking on all fours and finally crawled or wiggled her way into her brother's room. He was elated. We could hear him shouting, "I knew you could! You did great, Sis." And with that he gave her a big hug* (immediate, positive reinforcement). *Sis was smiling all over, obviously delighted with her brother's feedback.*

What motivation to change a behavior! When you begin to spark that same kind of enthusiasm in employees, just think of the things they will accomplish. The following are **Fine Points of Positive Feedback:***

---

*The fine points of positive and negative feedback are adapted from Blanchard, K. and Johnson, S.: The One Minute Manager. New York, William Morrow, 1982; also, Berkeley Books, 1986.

1. Catch employees doing things right. Remember, your job as a manager is to help employees succeed.

2. When employees are new on the job, remember to praise performance that is approximately right. This helps to guide their performance in the right direction. The reinforcement will help to make the appropriate behavior reappear and remain constant.

3. Make sure your nonverbal as well as verbal behavior clearly communicates to employees that you believe in them and feel good about their contributions to the organization.

Negative Feedback

Although positive feedback will help to keep employees moving straight ahead toward mutually agreed upon goals, there will be times when employees will get off course and adjustments will need to be made. In those instances, it is important to be able to give employees negative feedback. In an effort to soften the blow, many managers use the "sandwich approach" in giving negative feedback. They call employees in for a navigational adjustment and begin by giving them a compliment, followed by negative feedback, followed by another compliment. It might happen something like this:

Situation

The manager calls the employee into her office for the purpose of correcting her poor documentation of patient teaching.

Nurse Manager: **"Jane, you did a good job with Mr. Adams's dressing this morning, but you need to improve your documentation. I reviewed some of your charts last week, and your documentation is not complete enough in regard to patient teaching. Oh, by the way, I want you to know I really appreciate your being willing to work over this weekend."**

This feedback is too diluted to really have an impact. The manager started off with positive feedback and diluted it by immediately following it with a criticism. The criticism was also weakened by the immediate positive feedback that followed. When the sandwich approach is used repeatedly, the employee learns to dread every compliment, for fear that it is merely a set-up for a criticism.

The following **Fine Points of Negative Feedback** suggest an alternative to the sandwich approach.

1. Be very specific in telling an employee what she did wrong.
2. Let her know verbally and nonverbally how you feel about what she did wrong.
3. Pause and remain silent for a few seconds in order to let the employee feel your displeasure.
4. Verbally and nonverbally let the employee know that you value her and are on her side.
5. Make sure the employee understands that you are upset with her performance in this particular situation, but that you still think well of her.
6. Once you have given an employee the negative feedback, put it aside. Don't continue dwelling on it.

In the next example, the nurse manager gives the employee the same criticism using these fine points of negative feedback.

> *Manager:* **"Jane, I reviewed your charts this weekend, and I found that you need to improve your documentation of patient teaching. It is not enough to chart that you taught the patient. You need to give details about what you taught and the patient's reaction. I was disappointed to find your charting incomplete."** *(Pauses and touches Jane on the arm.)* **"Jane, I've seen you do a good job of teaching patients. I know you can also do a good job of documenting."**

CONCLUSION

As the manager, you are the captain of your ship. If you follow the general principles of giving feedback and incorporate the Fine Points of Positive and Negative Feedback, you will have mastered the art of keeping your crew on course. We wish you smooth sailing.

CREATIVE TEACHING TIPS

1. Form groups of three and practice giving each other positive feedback regarding a compliment from a doctor. Use the Fine Points of Positive Feedback. The third member of the group will serve as a coach.

2. In the same group of three, practice giving negative feedback regarding documentation using the Fine Points of Negative Feedback.

Putting It All Together

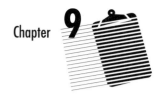

Clinical Skills Versus Management Skills:
With Everything Else You Have to Do, Why Would You Adopt a Monkey?

You are now familiar with the essential skills that will make you a more effective manager. You have a definition of an assertive manager and, through positive self-talk and imaging, you can see yourself moving in that direction. You have more than just the mental picture of yourself as an assertive manager. You know the skills involved in assertive communication. You have the tools to effectively manage stress, and you know how to invest your time wisely. You set goals with employees and give them feedback that can keep them motivated and moving toward better performance.

Your confidence as a manager will increase as you become more and more skillful in expressing yourself assertively. Employees will be more satisfied and thus more productive, and you will gain the respect of both management and staff. You will not always get exactly what you want from others, but because you are assertive, you will have the satisfaction of knowing that you have made your best effort.

THE MONKEY TRAP

Even with all this knowledge and skill, you are at risk because you are a health care manager. Your previous training, experience, and possibly even your personality traits all make you particularly vulnerable to be caught in a "monkey trap."* That is the trap you fall into each time you take on a

---

*The "monkey concept" is adapted from Blanchard, K., Oncken, W., Jr., and Burrows, H.: The One Minute Manager Meets the Monkey. New York, William Morrow, 1989.

responsibility (monkey) that belongs to an employee. You have adopted your employee's monkey.

As mentioned previously, most health care managers have training and experience in managing patients but do not have formal training in managing employees. When a health care worker is put into an unfamiliar situation and is asked to function, she will call upon familiar skills and apply them as best she can. Clinical skills, however, are different from management skills. It is the attempt to apply clinical skills to the management situation that can trap you unaware into the adoption of monkeys.

The health care worker's primary role is to meet the needs of the patient. The manager's primary role is to meet the needs of the organization by helping employees reach their full potential. The trap for the manager begins with her training and ability to empathize. Empathy, while a necessary skill in caring for patients and certainly helpful in relating to employees, can interfere with the health care manager's ability to manage. It is so easy to feel guilty when you can't solve employees' problems or when you have to ask employees to do something in spite of their problems.

Every time you do something for an employee that she can do for herself, you rescue her. When you take the "next move" that is rightfully hers, you have adopted her monkey. With adoption goes responsibility. Now the monkey is yours to feed and to care for. Interestingly, now that you have adopted her monkey, the employee becomes your supervisor, stopping by from time to time to see how well you are taking care of your (her) responsibility. You already have your own monkeys to care for (your responsibilities as a manager). If you fall into the monkey trap, you may find yourself adopting many monkeys and doing a poor job of tending to your own. Even more important to realize is that by adopting the employee's monkey you are interfering with her right to benefit the organization and to reach her full potential.

Avoiding the Monkey Trap

How can you successfully avoid the monkey trap? How can you manage so that every employee knows her own monkeys (job expectations) and is responsible for their care and feeding? When an employee offers her monkey for adoption, you have two alternatives depending on the nature of the problems the employee is having. You first determine if the employee *can do* or *can't do.**

---

*Adapted from Blanchard, K. and Lorber, R.: Putting the One Minute Manager to Work. New York, William Morrow, 1984, p 33.

Can Do

If the employee knows her responsibility and has the necessary knowledge and skill to perform but for some reason is not performing, you, as her manager, need to assume a supportive leadership style. Be understanding and talk about her alternatives. You may go back to the goals you have mutually set and give her feedback regarding her performance. After talking with you, the employee leaves with a clear understanding of what is expected and has some ideas as to how to solve her problems. Above all, she takes her monkey with her. *The next move is hers.*

Situation

A new health care manager is in conference with a staff nurse who is several years her senior, in both age and work experience.

Health Care Manager: Mary, I've noticed that you are late every morning. During the month I've been here, you've consistently come in 10 to 15 minutes after report has begun.

Staff Nurse (cheerfully): I've always come in at 7:45. You're so new, I guess you didn't know. I live far away and have to drop off my granddaughter at school. Everyone knows I do that. It's no problem. They all give me report later (starts to leave).

Health Care Manager: It's possible that I have some different expectations than your previous manager did. It's important to me to get things started on time. I like to have time to help staff set goals for the day and discuss problem areas.

Staff Nurse: It's always been fine and I just don't see how I can get here any earlier. If you want me to give up my break, I will.

Health Care Manager: I understand that it will involve rearranging your personal schedule, but I do expect you to get here on time. When you arrive late, it is disruptive and does not set a good example for others, and frankly I have felt very annoyed each time it has happened. *(Pauses and touches Mary's arm.)* As one of the senior employees on the unit, Mary, you are someone I count on to be a good role model for the younger nurses. Coming in late is not typical of your otherwise excellent performance. Because of your experience,

I had hoped to count on your help in making the daily assignments. It's very important to me that you be on time.

Staff Nurse: I didn't realize it was such a big deal. I guess I'll have to do something about it. Do you have any suggestions?

Health Care Manager: You might check with Sue. She has a similar situation. Let's decide when you can have the arrangements made. (Employee keeps her own monkey.)

Staff Nurse: Not tomorrow, for sure!

Health Care Manager: I understand. Let's see, today is Monday. How about Friday? Would that give you enough time to make arrangements?

Staff Nurse: I guess so.

Health Care Manager: So that we'll both be aware of your progress in this area, starting Friday I would like you to make a note of your arrival time every day. Let's plan to meet briefly next Wednesday to see how you're doing.

Staff Nurse: Okay.

*   *   *

Staff Nurse: It's Friday and here I am at 7:25!

Health Care Manager: Why, you're the first one here! I want to tell you how good I feel about that. I know it has taken some effort to rearrange your schedule, and I appreciate it. The unit is really going to benefit from your input in planning each morning. Since you're here first, why don't you go ahead and pick your lunch time.

Staff Nurse: Great!

Can't Do

You may determine, however, that an employee is having a *can't do* problem. She does not clearly understand her responsibilities, she has a different understanding of her responsibilities than you do, or she lacks the knowledge or skill to perform her responsibilities as expected. As the manager, you now assume a teaching/directive leadership style in which you may clarify goals and responsibilities, teach skills, and observe performance. There is an advantage to employees in being slow learners. If they wear you down to the point that you become impatient, you may weaken and decide that it would be easier to adopt the monkey.

> *New Graduate Nurse:* **I've been assigned Ms. Lopez today. I've never done tracheotomy care. Somebody else will have to do that. Will someone do it for me?**
>
> *Health Care Manager:* **It's important that you learn tracheotomy care. How can you best learn it?**
>
> *New Graduate Nurse:* **Well, I've watched Claire do tracheotomy care. I think if she helped me once or twice, I could do it.**
>
> *Health Care Manager:* **Good. I'll assign Claire to help you today and observe you tomorrow. At the end of the shift tomorrow we'll all three determine if you will need any further assistance with tracheotomy care.** (Employee keeps her own monkey.)
>
> *New Graduate Nurse:* **That sounds good.**

CONCLUSION

Health care teams develop patient care plans, based on the patient's needs and goals. Assertive managers work with employees to develop plans that are designed to meet the organization's goals and to assist employees in reaching their own full potential. The organization does not exist to meet the needs of employees; employees are hired to meet the needs of the organization. Although some employees can assume more responsibility than others, there is a minimum expectation of all. *An efficient, productive health care organization is one in which all monkeys are attended to regularly and promptly by their rightful owners.*

CREATIVE TEACHING TIPS
1. Using toy monkeys, develop a role play demonstrating the hazards of adopting monkeys and the assertive techniques for not adopting monkeys.
2. Using Appendix VI, identify a monkey that you will stop adopting. Pair up and practice not adopting this monkey.

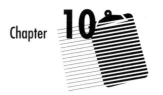

Customer Relations:
Just Looking for a Little Respect

Customers are anyone for whom you provide a service. In your role as a manager, your customers are your patients, patients' families, staff under your supervision, other hospital departments, other professionals providing service to the patient, and other agencies contracted to provide services. In the final analysis, customer relations is an employee relations issue, and the "buck stops" squarely with the manager. The health care manager has a twofold responsibility for customer service: (1) the delivery of excellent patient care and (2) the creation of gratified customers.

In today's health care environment, the manager is faced with the challenge of appropriate and safe patient care delegation. Today's manager may find herself responsible for a variety of personnel, both nursing and non-nursing, licensed and unlicensed. This responsibility requires that the manager be aware of the level of skill required for a task, the competency of the individual to whom the task is to be delegated, the job description of that person, and governing policies of the organization. Even though the manager delegates a task, she is still ultimately responsible for the safe performance of that task.

Creating an atmosphere of respect leads to gratified customers. The manager sets off a chain reaction by treating employees respectfully. The employees, in turn, will pass on this respect to others. In other words, employees will "Do unto others as they have been done to." The components of a **R-E-S-P-E-C-T-F-U-L** management style are as follows:

Reality: The reality is that customers are the reason for your existence. As obvious as it may seem, sometimes managers need to be reminded that without employees there would be no need for a manager. Staff may need to be reminded that without patients there would be no need for their services. Keeping this reality in focus helps maintain a positive attitude.

Empathy: Reflecting on personal experiences will increase your understanding of your customer's situation. Put yourself on the same feeling level with the customer and try to see a situation from the customer's perspective.

Self-Esteem: Helping someone maintain his or her identity increases that person's self-esteem. All your customers have a name, an identity, and a life. Show that you value your customers by taking the time to learn who they are.

Possibilities: Help customers find creative alternatives to potentially negative situations. De-emphasize what you can't do and emphasize what you can do for your customers. Help people identify their own strengths and assets.

Empowerment: Customers become empowered when they have information. Having information allows customers to be active partners. When customers participate in a process, they are more apt to be gratified with the results.

Customizing: Customers come to you with individual needs. Cookie-cutter, one-size-fits-all solutions are dehumanizing. The customer may not complain, but he or she is not gratified. Solutions that are tailor-made enhance the customer's gratification.

Touch: Providing gratifying customer service depends on how well you're able to stay in touch. Did the service you provided have the desired effect? Look for creative ways to follow up with individual customers. What satisfies customers today may not satisfy them tomorrow. Stay in touch with the changing needs of your customers.

Fun: A sense of humor can defuse anger, reduce stress, banish boredom, and create a more positive atmosphere. You can create a more gratifying experience for your customers if you learn to use humor professionally and sensitively.

Unexpected: Provide more than the customer expects. Anticipate the customer's needs. In the era of competitive health care, the little things make an experience memorable and gratify customers. When the staff you supervise freely go the extra mile with customers, this effort is a positive reflection on your managing style.

Legend: Customers will tell others about their experiences with your health care facility. Gratified customers will tell positive stories, thereby creating a living legend of excellence in customer relations.

The secret to gratified customers is **RESPECTFUL** customer service, and **RESPECTFUL** customer service begins with **you.**

CREATIVE TEACHING TIPS
1. Ask how many people know the name of internal customers such as the housekeeper, the mail carrier, the food service worker, and so forth in their work areas.
2. Implement Being A Good Finder (Appendix VII).

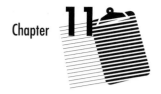

Chapter 11

Playing the Change Game:
The Process, the Players, the Practice

In today's competitive health care business, the name of the game is *change*. The only thing certain about health care today is that it won't be the same tomorrow. Capitation, corporatization, downsizing, rightsizing, restructuring, redesigning, re-engineering, and multiskilling are terms that reflect broad changes in health care delivery. Those who survive and thrive in the midst of this unpredictable environment will be those who learn to play the *Change Game*. As a manager, you will need to understand the change process and the impact it has on your staff. You will also need to recognize individual differences among your staff so that you can minimize their concerns and maximize their strengths. As the coach/advocate of your staff, you can help them change and grow through the process.

HOW THE GAME IS PLAYED

The *Change Game* involves losses. Health care providers who are unable or unwilling to change will be losers in the *Change Game*. Those who change will also experience loss—the loss of the familiar. Even when a situation is uncomfortable or ineffective, people often hang on to known problems rather than risk unknown solutions. Experiencing these losses associated with change triggers a process of grieving, as described by Kübler-Ross.* It is important that you understand the staff's needs and your role in each stage of the grief process.

Stage 1. Denial Resistance to the change is maximum. Shock, disbelief, and anxiety are prevalent emotions. During this stage people need time to

---

*Adapted from Kübler-Ross, E.: On Death and Dying. New York, Macmillan Publishing Co., Inc., 1969.

absorb the impact of the change. The staff needs an accepting, understanding attitude from the manager.

Stage 2. Anger   At this stage the employees are looking for something or someone to blame. If you recognize that their anger is directed at the perceived cause of the loss, it will help you understand and not personalize their anger. Remain nonjudgmental and allow people to ventilate. By staying focused, keeping your perspective, and remaining consistent with your message, you will see the staff's anxiety and anger begin to diminish.

Stage 3. Bargaining   This stage is an attempt to avoid the change. Staff will make promises and will try to negotiate deals in an effort to prevent or to delay the change. During this stage, the manager needs to be empathetic and patient. It is important to remain consistent regarding the reality of the change.

Stage 4. Depression   At this stage the full impact of the loss begins to set in. The staff may feel overwhelmed, hopeless, helpless, and powerless. Recognize that in this stage, people are looking for something to hold on to. Provide the staff with information only as they are ready to hear it. Recognize that problem-solving skills will be low during this stage. Information needs to be simple (written and verbal), with ample opportunity for questions.

Stage 5. Acceptance and Implementation   This is the problem-solving stage. The staff are now ready to move forward, and they are most receptive to new ideas. They are ready to become active participants in implementing the change. This is the optimum time to provide information and outside support. Bring in administrative personnel to discuss the change.

It is important to realize that grief, although described in five stages, is actually a very fluid process with movement in both directions. Response to change and progression through the grief process are highly individualized, largely due to the significance of the loss to the person involved and their investment in the current mode of operation.

THE PLAYERS IN THE GAME

If people were like pieces of furniture, change would be easy. People have personalities, however, and when faced with change, every personality responds differently. As the manager, you must take into consideration these differences in order to help each staff member move, contribute, and grow through the process. Just as it helps to understand grief by looking at it in five separate stages, it is also helpful to look at four personality types and the way each type responds to change.*

Think about each member of your staff as you read descriptions of the following personality types. No staff member will be a perfect fit, but each staff member will probably most resemble one type.

The Cheerleaders: These staff members are enthusiastic and energetic. They inspire others and ensure that the group has fun.

The Conductors: They are goal- and action-oriented. They are leaders, with the ability to motivate and to involve others.

The Critiquers: These staff members are perfectionists with high standards. They are orderly, are organized, and give attention to detail.

The Conciliators: They are competent negotiators. They like peace and harmony, and they have a knack for keeping things simple.

As these staff members are confronted with change, they move through the five stages of grief at their own rates and in their own styles. In grief stages 1, 2, 3, and 4, their views of their perceived losses explain their resistance to the change. In grief stage 5, their strengths provide resources to help themselves and others accept and implement the change (see Chart on next page).

But what about you? As the coach of your team, you are not exempt from grief as you face losses brought on by change. It is of utmost importance that you stay aware of your own feelings and work hard not to let your own reactions impede or negatively influence the implementation of the change. Which personality type best fits you? Recognize your reasons for resistance and maximize your positive influence by using your own best resources. Use your manager and your peers to help you be more objective in this self-analysis.

HOW TO WIN THE CHANGE GAME:
PRACTICE, PRACTICE, PRACTICE!

Winning the *Change Game* can be defined as successfully implementing changes. Successful implementation will result in improved health care

---

*Adapted from Littauer, F.: Personality Plus. Grand Rapids, MI, Fleming H. Revell, Revised, 1992.

Change: Reactions and Resources		
	REASONS FOR RESISTANCE: GRIEF STAGES 1, 2, 3, AND 4	UTILIZING STRENGTHS: GRIEF STAGE 5
CHEERLEADERS	• No fun • Too many new rules and regulations • Loss of special "star status"	• They are born promoters. Involve them in thinking of creative ways to "sell" the positive aspects of the change. • Challenge them to come up with group and individual rewards and incentives.
CONDUCTORS	• Loss of control • Loss of appreciation and credit for accomplishments • Fear of failure	• It is important that these leaders support the change. Ask for their help. • Give them responsibility. Put them in charge of task forces to implement change.
CRITIQUERS	• Disruption of schedule • Unknowns and risks • Uncertainty and unpredictability	• They are creative problem solvers. Utilize their abilities to organize, to schedule, and to work on the fine details of the change. • Use their artistic ability to make posters, bulletin boards, and newsletters.
CONCILIATORS	• Chaos and pressure • Conflict among the group • A lot of hard work	• Utilize their ability to be sensitive to the feelings of others. They can facilitate group discussions, mediate problems, and avoid or resolve conflict. • They can simplify the complicated and communicate it well.

delivery, a more cohesive staff, and team members who have been able to innovate and to grow as individuals through the process.

As the manager, you are responsible for creating an environment where innovation and change are the expected protocol. If small changes are implemented frequently, you can prevent stagnation and mental stenosis from afflicting you and your staff. If you keep exercising your change muscles, you will remain flexible, alert, creative, and self-confident. Smaller changes will be practice skirmishes for the inevitable big *Change Game* that will come along.

You can develop this dynamic environment and keep yourself and your staff in shape by remembering **C-H-A-N-G-E.**

Celebrate: Recognize and memorialize significant people and events. Even though things change and people leave, it is important to recognize their contributions. Celebrate the coming of new people and the implementation of change.

Horizons: Broaden the staff's horizons by encouraging them to attend workshops and professional meetings.

Axe: Axe rumors and misinformation. Ask staff members to check out rumors before spreading them to someone else. Freely share accurate information regarding changes with employees.

New: Encourage and reward staff members who find innovative ways to accomplish old tasks.

Grow: Expect the staff to grow by learning something new every day: a new medication, a new diagnosis, a new treatment, the name of a new customer, and so forth.

Exposure: Encourage sharing of newspaper articles, journal articles, and posters so that the employees are exposed to changes in health care delivery, technology, and customer relations.

Your job as manager will be to help staff members contribute to the initiation of change. When their ideas are implemented, they feel like participants in change rather than victims of change. Keep staff up to date and well informed. A knowledgeable staff will be prepared and powerful. As you are successful in creating this exciting atmosphere, you have laid the foundation for winning at any *Change Game* that may come your way.

CREATIVE TEACHING TIPS
1. Identify an anticipated change and brainstorm methods of support for each stage of the grief process.
2. Share stories regarding the successful implementation of change.

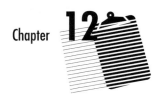

Chapter 12

Networking:
What Counts Is Not What You Know, But Who You Know Who Knows What You Need to Know

Within the formal structure of every organization there is an informal network. It is to your advantage as a health care manager to understand networking and to be able to identify, to utilize, and even to create informal networks.

GENERAL BENEFITS OF NETWORKING

John Naisbitt, in his 1982 classic *Megatrends,* defines networking as a process of "people talking to each other, sharing ideas, information and resources." As our society becomes more technologic and our knowledge becomes broader, we are all called upon to become more specialized and to find ways of sharing and communicating our special areas of knowledge with each other. As workers in health care have become more independent in their areas of expertise, they have become more dependent on co-workers who are experts in other areas.

In a network every person is important. Workers have an opportunity to make valuable contributions and to feel of value to the organization. Building good working relationships becomes of utmost importance because in the network management structure, management and workers are interdependent. Individual and organizational success depends upon the quality of the relationships. When networking works well, the organization becomes warm, friendly, and family-like rather than cold and impersonal.

In *Megatrends 2000,* Naisbitt and Aburdene observe that today's worker places personal growth as a higher priority than company loyalty. Members of the new workforce will help your organization achieve its objectives if they can achieve their own personal goals as part of the bargain. Today's health care workers know that in the face of rapidly changing organizations, they need to be creatively growing, developing, and making contacts that will be of benefit to them in their careers. Although it may seem contradictory, it is our belief that employees will be loyal to the organization that is helping and encouraging them to outgrow their current jobs.

The organization benefits from networking. Workers who feel that they are able to make valuable contributions will be happier and more productive. Because workers are encouraged to cut through traditional chains of command and to go directly to the source of needed information, work is performed more efficiently and effectively. Networks can go beyond sharing information to the creation of knowledge. Each person in a network takes in new information and creates other new ideas.

We have all experienced the energy and creativity that can be generated when individuals are brought together in a think-tank or brainstorming situation. The outcome is usually a list of ideas of superior quantity and quality than all the individuals could have generated had they worked separately. Another positive outcome is the camaraderie that develops among group members as they stimulate each other's creativity. In Stephen Covey's *The Seven Habits of Highly Effective People,* he describes this phenomenon as synergy.

ADVANTAGES OF NETWORKING FOR HEALTH CARE MANAGERS

In your role as manager, you are a member of a multidisciplinary team. You can readily utilize the concept of networking if you understand the value of shared knowledge and realize that there is strength in numbers. The manager who attempts to be self-sufficient and all-knowing today is working *hard.* The manager who works *smart* learns that the important thing is not what you know, but who you know who knows what you need to know. A successful health care manager today will develop her networking abilities and will teach these skills to the staff.

When you utilize the networking process, you do not have to be the most knowledgeable clinician on your unit. Your goal, in fact, will be to develop staff members who are more knowledgeable in certain areas than you are. Your challenge is to create a work environment where individuals of diverse skills and interests can grow in their own unique ways. At the same time, you need to provide enough structure so that the collective efforts of all will benefit the organization. Benefits resulting from the networking process are as follows:

1. Information of increased variety and depth is available to the staff.
2. Information is more accessible to the staff.
3. Each staff member has an opportunity to make a more valuable contribution to the organization.
4. Each staff member can pursue an individual area of interest.
5. Patients receive better care because all staff members are kept up-to-date on new information.
6. Team spirit is enhanced by creating a team of health care experts, each of whom is making a valuable contribution, while relying on each other for information and assistance.
7. Interested staff members have an opportunity to assume more responsibility and to excel beyond the minimal expectations of their jobs.
8. High energy, creativity, and innovation are created, thus promoting a positive and exciting work environment.

The following is an example of a nurse manager's goal and plan to establish a network of nursing experts on her unit in a large hospital.

Goal-Setting Worksheet

Date Today

Desired Outcome: Unit 5 North will develop a network of experts among R.N. staff. All staff members will choose and develop an area of interest that will be of benefit to them and the unit as a whole.

Deadline for Achievement* (One year from today)

Steps Toward Achievement	Intermediate Deadlines	Name of Person or Group Responsible
1. Each R.N. chooses an area and submits it to the nurse manager, who will review and negotiate possible duplications.	(1 month from today)	Each R.N., nurse manager

Steps Toward Achievement	Intermediate Deadlines	Name of Person or Group Responsible
2. A schedule of unit inservice programs will be developed so that each R.N. will make a 30-minute presentation of her area of interest within the coming calendar year.	(1 month from today)	Nurse manager
3. Each R.N. will be encouraged to attend a workshop or training session in her area of interest this year. Tuition assistance will be requested from the Medical Center.	(1 year from today)	Each R.N., nurse manager, director of continuing education
4. Each R.N. will provide the unit with current information (from journal articles and books) in her area of interest.	(1 year from today)	Each R.N.
5. Each R.N. will serve as a consultant to other staff members on the unit regarding her area of interest.	Ongoing	Each R.N.
6. The nurse manager will be aware of each R.N.'s area of interest and will be responsible for connecting a nurse who has a need with the nurse who has the information.	Ongoing	Nurse manager

Date for Review, Revision, or Update		Name of Person or Group Responsible
(6 months from today)		Nurse manager

*Deadlines should be as specific as possible. Use actual dates.

CREATIVE TEACHING TIPS

1. Ask the participants to complete the Setting a Goal for Success sheet (Appendix VIII) and network to gather useful information for achieving their career goals.

2. Develop a list of experts from the group.

Chapter 13

Power:
It All Adds Up

What are your feelings about the word *power?* Is it a positive, comfortable concept for you, or does the mention of the word make you uneasy? As you examine your feelings, you may discover that, like many health care managers, you are ambivalent about power. In your head you know that having power is desirable, but in your heart you're not so sure. Your responses to the following statements will help you assess your reactions to power.

Reactions to Power

1. The desire for power is a normal, healthy emotion.   True ____ False ____

2. Power itself is neither good nor bad, but its use can be constructive or destructive.   True ____ False ____

3. It is possible to exert power without violating the rights of others.   True ____ False ____

4. Power is not a gender-related trait.   True ____ False ____

5. You cannot have a good self-image if you feel powerless.   True ____ False ____

6. Being an expert at using power is more important to the health care manager than being an expert clinician.   True ____ False ____

7. Health care workers often underestimate their power.   True ____ False ____

8. Power comes from realistically evaluating and using all your personal assets and legitimate authority.   True ____ False ____

9. In order to be effective, the health care
   manager must establish her own power base. True ___ False ___

10. Interpersonal alliances are helpful ways of
    acquiring power. True ___ False ___

11. Powerful people are rational thinkers. True ___ False ___

12. Feelings of helplessness lead to burnout. True ___ False ___

13. Power is necessary to bring about change. True ___ False ___

14. It is more profitable to negotiate a
    compromise from a position of power. True ___ False ___

15. The "goodies" (staff, equipment, money for
    continuing education) go to the people who
    are most visible. True ___ False ___

As you took the test, it must have been obvious that the appropriate answer to each question is "True." That was your intellectual reaction. Now read the test again, but this time try to become more aware of your emotional reaction. Do you equate power with negative behavior, such as intimidation and aggression? Can you acknowledge openly that having power is necessary for you to effectively perform your duties as a manager? Do you deny that having power is important, lest someone accuse you of being power-hungry? Can you honestly admit, without guilt or embarrassment, that the enjoyment of power has been a motivating influence in your advancement toward a management position?

You know you need power and you probably even want it, but you may be hesitant to acknowledge or use it. Your self-talk possibly sounds something like this: "Maybe I could have some power but not tell anyone. I could exert just a little power—enough to help me handle a problem employee, but not enough to offend anyone. I could be powerful but disguise it so that the staff wouldn't notice. They would just keep on treating me like one of the gang."

You have a responsibility to your organization and to those you manage to understand fully and to utilize the authority that has been delegated to you. The powerless cannot help the powerless. Employees need a powerful leader. Set a goal now to become more comfortable with the power that is rightfully and necessarily yours as a manager.

THREE COMPONENTS OF POWER

The idea of *power* may have a negative connotation until its components are examined. *Webster's New World Dictionary* defines power as "the ability to do, act, or produce . . .; legal ability or authority . . ." Power is the combination of three components: *authority, ability,* and *action.* When a manager who has been given *authority* to lead also possesses the *ability* to lead and then takes *action,* she is exercising power. Being given authority is like having a driver's license; it is the legal capacity to act. Possessing ability is the same as having a car with a full tank of gas; it is the capability for action. Until someone takes action, turns on the ignition, presses the accelerator, and guides the car, however, no one goes anywhere. Consider the following formulas:

Authority + Ability − Action = Impotent Manager
Authority + Action − Ability = Incompetent Manager
Action + Ability − Authority = Illegitimate Manager
Authority + Ability + Action = Powerful Assertive Manager

The impotent manager uses a passive management style. Because her goal is to avoid conflict, she avoids making decisions or taking decisive actions. By attempting to please employees, she relinquishes her power to the employees.

The incompetent manager lacks management skills such as goal setting, giving feedback, or managing time. She may not know how to avoid assuming responsibility for employees. She may not know how to communicate or to listen assertively. Her lack of ability in one or more of these areas results in increased stress and low job satisfaction for herself as well as for employees.

The illegitimate manager uses an aggressive management style. Her main concern is achieving results, and this need may lead her to do things her way rather than to follow prescribed policies and procedures. Any progress may be sacrificed in the long run because of the problems created. Her illegitimate actions will also result in increased stress and low job satisfaction for her and for employees.

A powerful leader combines the authority to act with the ability to act and to make things happen. When a manager takes legitimate effective action, both the manager and the employees benefit. The manager experiences less stress and greater job satisfaction. Employees feel more secure and are more productive and better satisfied. When a manager is assertive, everyone wins, including the organization and its customers.

EXAMPLES OF POWER

The following are examples of actions taken by powerful nurse managers:

1. A nurse manager negotiated with nursing administration to allow some employees to work the flexible time schedule that they requested.

2. A nurse manager informed a surgeon that one of the staff nurses had developed expertise in the physical and psychologic care of patients undergoing mastectomies. They arranged for the staff nurse to present an inservice program for the surgical residents, interns, and medical students.

3. A nurse manager, noticing the anxiety in the families of patients in the intensive care unit, arranged for two R.N.s, a social worker, and the hospital chaplain to plan a program to better meet the needs of these family members.

4. When a physician criticized an R.N. for overstepping her bounds by providing an unwed teenage mother information on birth control, the nurse manager defended the nurse's role as a health care educator.

5. After noticing that patients referred from a particular hospital were often unprepared for a visit from one of her nurses, the nurse manager of a home health care agency arranged a meeting with the director of nursing from that hospital to discuss the problem. The result was a research project to investigate whether patients who were prepared for the transition to home health care, according to a defined protocol, were less likely to be readmitted to the hospital.

6. When two R.N.s requested approval to attend a conference, but only one could be funded or spared from the unit, the nurse manager chose to approve attendance for the one whose written professional goals would be better met.

EMPOWERING EMPLOYEES

In the aggressive, authoritarian management style of the past, a manager would withhold information from employees as a way of maintaining control over them. The "boss" would say "jump," and the workers would not ask, "Why?" but would ask, "How high?" Today's workers will simply say, "Goodbye!" The better educated, more entrepreneurial health care workers want to feel in partnership with their employer. They want a manager who leads by example. They will respond to an empowering assertive style of leadership.

The assertive manager empowers employees by stating expectations and by giving positive and negative feedback regarding performance. She maintains two-way communication that is open, honest, and direct. Through freely and consistently sharing information and encouraging employees' self-development, the assertive manager facilitates employees' opportunities to benefit the organization and to reach their full potential.

The empowering manager operates using the following formula:

**Recognizes Ability + Delegates Authority + Rewards Action
= Empowered Employees**

CREATIVE TEACHING TIPS

1. Develop a role play to illustrate each of the five formulas.

2. The health care managers in your organization have been "accused of having power." Divide into two teams and have a mock trial, with one team arguing for the defense and one team arguing for the prosecution.

Appendix I

CHANGING "YOU" MESSAGES TO "I" MESSAGES

Instructions: Change the following "You" messages to "I" messages.

1. You never get to work on time.

2. You should have completed the charting on Mr. Jones.

3. You should have returned Dr. Smith's call like you said you would.

4. You said you taught Mrs. Williams how to test her urine, but that's not what she tells me.

5. You should have opened that new case yesterday.

6. You should have called back to the office before you went home so that this problem could have been avoided.

7. You should know how to order oxygen by now.

8. You should know that someone must work on the holiday.

Appendix II

THE SEVEN SECRETS OF STRESS MANAGEMENT

In order to reduce my stress, I endorse the following statements:

1. I *choose to believe* that each person is doing his or her best.
2. Expectation affects outcomes, so I *choose* to expect a positive outcome.
3. If I always do what I've always done, I'll always get what I've always gotten.
4. I can influence others, but only they can choose to change.
5. Life is not always fair.
6. Worry is more stressful than action.
7. I always have a *choice,* and all choices have consequences.

When faced with a stressful situation, I ask myself:

1. What am I telling myself about the situation?
2. Is my self-talk in my best interest?
3. Is this situation my business?
4. Do I have the power to change the situation?
5. What are the alternatives in this situation?
6. What are the consequences of my choice?
7. What can I do *now* to reduce my stress?

Appendix III

COMMITMENT TO REDUCE MY STRESS

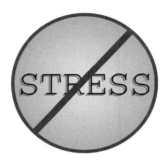

I promise to read the Seven Secrets of Stress Management three times a day for 21 days and to practice the secrets daily.

_____
Date

_____
Name

_____
Street or Apt.

_____
City   State   Zip

_____
Phone Number

Appendix IV

DISPUTING IRRATIONAL THINKING

Instructions: Read the following irrational statements and practice changing them to rational statements.

1. I should be able to answer all questions from my staff.

2. I must work hard all the time.

3. I must always come earlier and stay later than anyone on my staff.

4. It is awful when I make mistakes.

5. People should do things the right way (my way).

6. Goals should not be so hard to achieve.

7. I must finish work before I play.

8. People should treat me fairly.

9. A person who has reached my level should not make mistakes.

10. I can't stand it when people don't like something I've done.

11. My staff should follow my directions and do what I ask them to do.

12. Things should work out the way I want them to.

13. It is awful when my staff does not like a decision I have made.

14. I should always achieve my goals.

15. People should not get mad at me.

16. I should be able to solve my staff's problems.

17. I should be able to manage any crisis that comes up.

18. I should be able to get my work done on time.

19. If people in my area are dissatisfied, it is my fault.

20. It is awful when my supervisor gives me negative feedback.

Appendix V

GOAL-SETTING WORKSHEET

Date

Desired Outcome:

Deadline for Achievement:

Steps Toward Achievement	*Intermediate Deadlines*	*Name of Person or Group Responsible*

Date for Review, Revision, or Update	*Name of Person or Group Responsible*

Appendix VI

AVOIDING THE MONKEY TRAP

I choose to no longer accept responsibility for the following monkey:

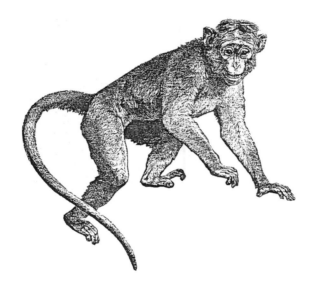

_____

_____

_____

Signature _____

Date _____

Appendix VII

BEING A GOOD FINDER

Instructions: Be a good finder. When you pan for gold, you have to sift through a lot of dirt before you find those precious nuggets. Your focus is not on the dirt you are sifting through but on the gold you are looking for. Treat yourself and others as if you're panning for gold. Stay focused on the good qualities in yourself and in others. Be a good finder and catch people doing good.

Good Findings

I caught . . .

1. someone interacting positively with a patient or a patient's family.

2. someone interacting positively with another staff member.

3. someone being enthusiastic about work.

4. someone being an encourager.

5. someone giving a patient positive feedback.

6. someone being supportive of change.

7. someone using humor in a healthy, constructive way.

8. someone going that extra mile by . . .

Appendix VIII

SETTING A GOAL FOR SUCCESS

What would I do within the next year to advance my career, if I knew I could not fail?

The Following Additional Questions Will Help You Set Your Goal for Success:

1. Can I visualize myself accomplishing this goal?
2. Is this a growth goal?
3. Am I willing to devote time, energy, and resources to achieve this goal?
4. Will this goal open doors of opportunity for me?
5. Can I get excited about this goal?

Appendix IX

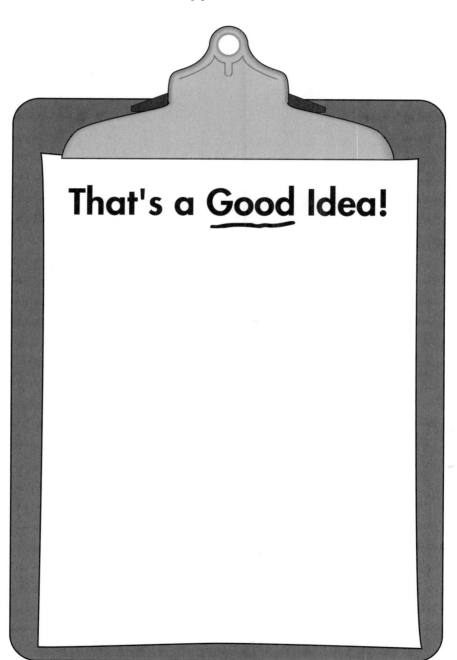

That's a <u>Good</u> Idea!

ANNOTATED BIBLIOGRAPHY

Current and classic references that have influenced our thinking and have helped us to develop our management philosophy

The American Nurses Association Staff Nurse Guide to Work Redesign. American Nurses Association, June 1995.
> *A comprehensive look at work redesign in the health care industry.*

The ANA Basic Guide To Safe Delegation. American Nurses Association, June 1995.
> *A flyer that outlines all the points that must be considered by a nurse manager before a task is delegated.*

Blanchard, K. and Bowles, S.: Raving Fans. New York, William Morrow, 1993.
> *In parable form, the fundamentals of moving customer service from simply preventing complaints to creating "raving fans."*

Blanchard, K. and Johnson, S.: The One Minute Manager. New York, William Morrow, 1982.
> *A practical step-by-step guide to goal-setting and feedback.*

Blanchard, K. and Lorber, R.: Putting the One Minute Manager to Work. New York, William Morrow, 1984.
> *Practical application of the secrets of one-minute goal-setting, one-minute praisings, and one-minute reprimands.*

Blanchard, K., Oncken, W., Jr., and Burrows, H.: The One Minute Manager Meets the Monkey. New York, William Morrow, 1989.
> *A story format that presents rules of "monkey management" to help harried, overwhelmed managers gain control of their lives.*

Covey, S.: The Seven Habits of Highly Effective People. New York, Simon and Schuster, 1989.
> *A principle-centered approach to improved interpersonal relations. Habit Six (Synergize) is especially helpful for team-building.*

Covey, S., Merrill, R. A., and Merrill, R. R.: First Things First: To Live, to Love, to Learn, to Leave a Legacy. New York, Simon and Schuster, 1994.
> *A principle-centered approach to time management that challenges our old paradigms.*

Ellis, A.: Reason and Emotion in Pyschotherapy. New York, Carol Publishing Group, Revised 1994.
> *Comprehensive work on rational emotive behavioral therapy. Clearly describes ABC's of emotion, rational and irrational thinking, and techniques for disputing irrational thinking.*

Kübler-Ross, E.: On Death and Dying. New York, Macmillan Publishing Co., Inc., 1969.
> *The original classic work on coping mechanisms during a time of loss and grief.*

Littauer, F.: Personality Plus. Grand Rapids, MI, Fleming H. Revell, Revised 1992.
> *A quick but amazingly accurate personality test and a detailed discussion of the strengths and weaknesses of each of the four personality types.*

Littauer, F. and Littauer, M.: Personality Puzzle: Understanding the People You Work With. Grand Rapids, MI, Fleming H. Revell, 1992.
> *The principles taught in Personality Plus applied to the workplace. Real-life situations and humorous anecdotes illustrate the uniqueness and value of each "piece of the puzzle."*

Naisbitt, J.: Megatrends. New York, Warner Books, 1982.
> *A classic work on how technology has changed society. An excellent chapter on networking.*

Naisbitt, J. and Aburdene, P.: Megatrends 2000. New York, William Morrow, 1990.
Insight into what motivates today's workers.

Smith, M.: When I Say No I Feel Guilty. New York, Bantam Books, 1975.
A classic work on assertive skills.

Ziglar, Z.: See You At The Top. Gretna, LA, Pelican, 1977.
A classic in motivational literature. Chapters on self-image, relationships, attitude, and work; an outstanding chapter and illustration on goal-setting.

Index

Note: Page numbers followed by the letter t refer to tables. An asterisk following a page number indicates that an application example is included.